Laboratory Manual for

Laboratory Procedures
for Veterinary Technicians

Laboratory Manual for

Laboratory Procedures for Veterinary Technicians

Seventh Edition

Margi Sirois, EdD, MS, RVT, CVT, LAT, VTES
Ashworth College
Norcross, Georgia

ELSEVIER

LABORATORY MANUAL FOR
LABORATORY PROCEDURES FOR VETERINARY TECHNICIANS,
SEVENTH EDITION

ISBN: 978-0-323-59540-7

Notice

Practitioners and researchers must always rely on their own experience and knowledge in evaluating and using any information, methods, compounds or experiments described herein. Because of rapid advances in the medical sciences, in particular, independent verification of diagnoses and drug dosages should be made. To the fullest extent of the law, no responsibility is assumed by Elsevier, authors, editors or contributors for any injury and/or damage to persons or property as a matter of products liability, negligence or otherwise, or from any use or operation of any methods, products, instructions, or ideas contained in the material herein.

Publishing Director: Kristin Wilhelm
Content Strategist: Brandi Graham
Senior Content Development Manager: Ellen Wurm-Cutter
Senior Content Development Editor: Maria Broeker
Publishing Services Manager: Shereen Jameel
Project Manager: Aparna Venkatachalam

Printed in India

Last digit is the print number: 9 8 7 6 5

ELSEVIER

3251 Riverport Lane
St. Louis, Missouri 63043

Working together to grow libraries in developing countries

www.elsevier.com • www.bookaid.org

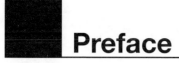

Preface

This laboratory manual is intended to accompany the seventh edition of *Laboratory Procedures for Veterinary Technicians*. Each unit in the laboratory manual relates to a corresponding unit in the textbook and stresses the essential information of the unit through the use of definitions, short essays (comprehension), photo quizzes, matching completion, word searches, and crossword puzzles.

Learning objectives are included at the beginning of each unit to help you focus on the material and concepts that you are expected to learn.

The following suggestions will help you use this laboratory manual to identify your strengths and weaknesses.

1. Review the contents of each unit before you attempt to do the exercises. Do not treat the questions individually and then refer to the text for the correct answer. Instead, deal with the unit's subject matter as a whole because many of the questions are interrelated. This is a learning exercise meant to help you learn the material presented in the textbook, not an examination for grades.

2. Read each question and study each illustration carefully before answering. You may know the answer or you may arrive at the correct answer by knowing which answers are incorrect.

3. The laboratory manual is designed so that the pages can be easily removed, submitted if required, and placed in your notebook with the corresponding lecture notes.

The answers to all exercises appear in the *Instructor Resources for Laboratory Procedures for Veterinary Technicians*, Seventh Edition, on the Evolve website at: http://evolve.elsevier.com/Sirois/vettech/.

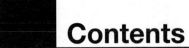

Contents

1 The Veterinary Practice Laboratory

LEARNING OBJECTIVES

When you have completed this unit, you should be able to:

1. Identify, use, and maintain personal protective equipment.

2. Describe the components of the Material Safety and Data Sheet (MSDS).

3. Create a label for a chemical container.

4. Differentiate between horizontal and angled head centrifuges.

5. Describe proper use and care of the centrifuge.

6. Discuss the selection and proper use of pipettes.

7. Calibrate a refractometer.

8. Identify the parts of a microscope.

9. List the steps in examining a microscope slide.

10. Demonstrate knowledge of basic mathematic principles.

11. Demonstrate understanding of metric and SI units.

12. Describe the components of a quality assurance program.

13. Differentiate between accuracy and precision.

14. Describe methods for verifying accuracy of test results.

EXERCISE 1.1: SAFETY AND OSHA STANDARDS

Instructions: Answer the following questions.

1. List the sections of the MSDS and the information that must be present on it.

_____

_____

_____

_____

_____

_____

_____

_____

_____

_____

_____

_____

_____

_____

2. Under what condition(s) do chemical containers require secondary labels?

_____

_____

_____

_____

3. Where are the following items located in your laboratory?

   a. Fire extinguisher

   _____

   b. MSDS binder

   _____

   c. Eye wash station

   _____

   d. Spill clean-up kit

   _____

4. List the types of personal protective equipment that are available in your laboratory.

_____

_____

_____

_____

EXERCISE 1.2: MATCHING: HAZARD SIGNS

Instructions: Match the hazard communicated with each of the pictograms.

1.

    a. Health hazard

2.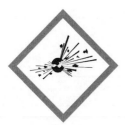

    b. Flammable

3.

    c. Acute toxicity

4.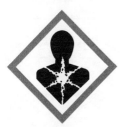

    d. Corrosion

5.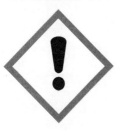

    e. Irritant

6.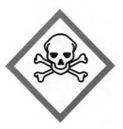

    f. Explosive

Chapter **1** **The Veterinary Practice Laboratory**

EXERCISE 1.3: DEFINING KEY TERMS

Instructions: Define each term in your own words.

1. Occupational Safety and Health Administration (OSHA)

   _____

   _____

2. Biohazard

   _____

   _____

3. Engineering controls

   _____

   _____

4. Personal protective equipment

   _____

   _____

5. Chemical hygiene plan

   _____

   _____

EXERCISE 1.4: LABORATORY EXERCISE: SECONDARY CONTAINER LABELING

Procedure:

1. Locate the MSDS binder.

2. Choose a chemical that is supplied in bulk (e.g., isopropyl alcohol).

3. Complete the sample label with the correct information.

Product Identifier Code _____ Product Name _____	**Hazard Pictograms**
	Signal Word
Supplier Information Company name _____ Address _____ _____ Emergency Phone Number _____	**Hazard Statements**
	Supplemental Information

Instructions: Find the words that are defined by the clues given below. The words may be located horizontally, vertically, or diagonally and may be reversed.

```
M  D  W  U  Z  O  O  N  O  S  E  S  K  M  L

F  S  E  J  P  X  E  R  P  C  X  Y  B  A  S

Z  E  D  H  Q  G  R  W  I  A  E  C  O  R  H

N  Y  Z  S  O  O  Q  B  M  G  U  Y  K  G  Q

D  Y  W  H  V  B  S  P  T  H  L  J  M  O  B

K  R  T  W  E  T  D  R  Y  Z  F  M  Z  T  U

D  A  A  E  N  R  O  B  D  O  O  L  B  C  X

P  K  U  Z  R  B  X  R  E  E  V  C  I  I  M

R  P  E  I  A  L  V  D  N  P  F  S  D  P  E

N  X  G  O  Z  H  C  L  B  H  Y  V  N  P  I

U  P  S  U  O  Z  O  O  J  X  C  V  Z  A  W

L  H  N  H  P  W  X  I  T  W  O  N  Y  M  L

A  V  H  S  C  F  Q  R  B  E  P  P  K  W  Y

C  O  L  G  F  D  I  E  A  J  R  C  T  B  I

E  L  F  I  H  C  H  G  I  S  O  H  Q  U  W
```

BIOHAZARD   PATHOGEN
BLOODBORNE   PICTOGRAM
MSDS   PPE
OPIM   ZOONOSES
OSHA

EXERCISE 1.6: GENERAL LABORATORY EQUIPMENT

Instructions: Answer the following questions.

1. Differentiate between fixed and angled head centrifuges. Which type is present in your laboratory?

   _____

   _____

   _____

   _____

2. Which type of pipette is used to add small volumes to another liquid and must be rinsed with the second liquid and the fluid remaining in the tip blown out?

   _____

3. List the type of temperature-controlled equipment in your laboratory, and state the normal range of operating temperatures for this equipment.

   _____

   _____

   _____

   _____

4. Which of the following images depicts a properly balanced centrifuge?

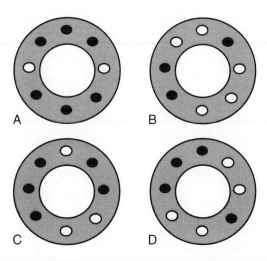

5. What do the scales inside the refractometer represent?

_____

_____

_____

_____

EXERCISE 1.7: DEFINING KEY TERMS

Instructions: Define each term in your own words.

1. Supernatant

_____

2. Refractive index

_____

_____

EXERCISE 1.8: LABORATORY EXERCISE: REFRACTOMETER CALIBRATION

Procedure:

1. Inspect and clean the prism cover glass and cover plate.

2. Place 1 drop of distilled water on the prism cover glass and close the cover.

3. Point the refractometer toward bright artificial light or sunlight.

4. Bring the light–dark boundary line into focus by turning the eyepiece.

5. Read and record the result with the specific gravity scale.

Result _____

6. If the refractometer does not provide a reading of 1.000, turn the set screw until the reading is correct.

7. Clean the refractometer according to the manufacturer's recommendations.

EXERCISE 1.9: LABORATORY EXERCISE: CENTRIFUGE CALIBRATION

Procedure:

1. Run the centrifuge for 3 to 5 minutes. Use a stopwatch to verify that the centrifuge remains running for the time chosen.

2. If available, use a tachometer to verify that the centrifuge is reaching the speed chosen. (NOTE: Do not perform this verification unless the centrifuge head can be viewed while closed!)

EXERCISE 1.10: WORD SEARCH: LABORATORY EQUIPMENT

Find the words that are defined by the clues given below. The words may be located horizontally, vertically, or diagonally and may be reversed.

```
P  E  Q  H  D  I  D  H  A  L  N  H  C  A  X
R  E  F  R  A  C  T  O  M  E  T  E  R  E  C
A  P  I  P  E  T  T  E  M  A  V  S  D  R  O
C  L  L  H  H  G  O  I  B  K  U  N  P  O  N
T  J  I  P  K  I  R  R  X  P  I  E  H  T  I
G  Z  J  Q  M  P  E  N  E  E  S  C  E  A  C
N  O  F  Y  U  T  F  R  V  U  S  H  D  B  A
O  J  V  D  A  O  N  I  O  I  G  G  N  U  L
S  F  D  W  Y  A  T  O  U  H  W  U  D  C  T
G  I  W  D  T  C  B  M  O  D  P  F  Y  N  U
Y  N  K  A  A  S  T  T  I  Z  K  L  R  I  B
M  D  N  R  Y  N  G  I  F  X  K  O  S  K  E
D  T  F  W  N  B  Z  G  Z  Z  E  Q  I  X  S
Z  E  G  U  F  I  R  T  N  E  C  R  R  E  R
R  C  E  M  P  X  I  J  D  G  U  U  S  B  U
```

ALIQUOTMIXER	REFRACTIVEINDEX
CENTRIFUGE	REFRACTOMETER
CONICALTUBES	SUPERNATANT
INCUBATOR	WATERBATH
PIPETTE	

EXERCISE 1.11: MICROSCOPE PARTS

Instructions: Answer the following questions.

1. Another name for flat-field objective lenses is _____.

2. The _____ on the microscope serves to aim and focus the light through the specimen.

3. To obtain the final magnification of an object, multiply the magnifications of the _____ lens and the _____ lens.

4. Excess oil may require the use of the chemical _____ for cleaning.

EXERCISE 1.12: PHOTO QUIZ: LABEL THE PARTS OF THE MICROSCOPE

Instructions: Label each microscope part.

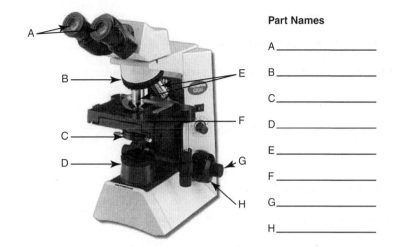

Part Names

A _____

B _____

C _____

D _____

E _____

F _____

G _____

H _____

EXERCISE 1.13: LABORATORY EXERCISE: CALIBRATING THE MICROSCOPE

Procedure:

1. Start at low power (10×) and focus on the 2-mm line if using the stage micrometer. The 2-mm mark equals 2000 μm.

2. Rotate the ocular micrometer within the eyepiece so that its hatchmark scale is horizontal and parallel to the stage micrometer.

3. Align the 0 points on both scales.

4. Determine the point on the stage micrometer aligned with the 10 hatchmark on the ocular micrometer.

5. Multiply this number by 100. In this example, 0.100 × 100 = 10 μm. This means that at this power (10×), the distance between each hatchmark on the ocular micrometer is 10 μm. Any object may be measured with the ocular micrometer scale, and that distance is measured by multiplying the number of ocular units by a factor of 10. For example, if an object is 10 ocular units long, then its true length is 100 μm (10 ocular units × 10 μm = 100 μm).

6. Repeat this procedure at each magnification.

7. For each magnification, record this information, and label it on the base of the microscope for future reference. The ocular micrometer within the microscope is now calibrated for the duration.
   Objective distance between hatchmarks (micrometers):
   4×:
   10×:
   40×:

11

EXERCISE 1.14: LABORATORY EXERCISE: USING THE COMPOUND LIGHT MICROSCOPE

Procedure:

1. Obtain a prepared microscope slide.

2. Clean the ocular and objective lenses with lens tissue.

3. Use the coarse adjustment knob to raise the nosepiece to its highest position.

4. Raise the condenser to its highest position.

5. Rotate the turret to move the scanning lens into position.

6. Turn on the microscope light.

7. Open the diaphragm to allow maximum light through the condenser.

8. Place the slide on the microscope stage, and secure it with the stage clips.

9. Look through the oculars and adjust the interpupillary distance so that one image is seen.

10. Look through the oculars and use the coarse adjustment knob to bring the slide into focus.

11. Use the fine adjustment to bring the slide into sharp focus.

12. If necessary, perform Köhler illumination adjustment (see below).

13. Use the stage controls to scan the entire slide while looking through the oculars.

14. Choose an object from the slide, center it in the field of view, and ensure that it is in sharp focus.

15. Rotate the turret to move the low-power objective into place.

16. Refocus the slide using, first, the coarse adjustment knob and then the fine adjustment knob.

17. Rotate the turret to move the high-power objective into place.

18. Refocus the slide by using *only* the fine adjustment knob.

19. Scan the slide by using the stage controls.

20. Rotate the turret so that the oil immersion objective is to the side (no objective is directly over the slide).

21. Place 1 drop of immersion oil on the center of the slide.

22. Rotate the turret to place the oil immersion lens into position over the slide. Ensure that the high-power objective does not come into contact with the oil and that the oil immersion lens is touching the drop of oil.

23. Refocus the slide by using *only* the fine adjustment knob.

24. Scan the slide.

25. When finished, rotate the turret to put the scanning lens in position over the slide.

26. Remove the slide from the stage, and gently wipe away the oil on the slide.

27. Wipe the oculars and the scanning, low-power, and high-power lenses by using lens tissue.

28. Use lens tissue to wipe the oil from the oil immersion lens.

29. Turn off the microscope.

30. Use the coarse adjustment knob to position the nosepiece to its lowest position.

31. Center the stage so that it is not protruding on either side of the microscope.

32. Cover the microscope with a dust cover.

Adjusting the Microscope for Köhler Illumination

1. Secure a slide on the microscope stage.

2. Adjust the light source to approximately half its total brightness.

3. Place the 10× ocular lens in position.

4. Verify that the eyepiece is at the correct interpupillary distance and the eyepiece is focused.

5. Focus on the specimen by using the coarse adjustment knob.

6. Close the field diaphragm and condenser until a small ring of light is visible in the field of view through the specimen.

7. If needed, adjust the condenser screws until the light is centered in the field of view.

8. Open the diaphragm until the circle of light just touches the edge of the circumference of the field of view.

9. Adjust the condenser until the light is in sharp focus. This may make the image darker, so adjust the brightness to compensate.

10. Repeat the procedure for each of the ocular objectives.

EXERCISE 1.15: WORD SEARCH: MICROSCOPY

Instructions: Find the words that are defined by the clues given below. The words may be located horizontally, vertically, or diagonally and may be reversed.

```
B  R  P  A  T  B  N  T  G  Q  M  Y  W  C  S
N  A  Z  I  L  V  F  N  F  U  W  Z  I  R  E
F  L  U  O  R  E  S  C  E  N  T  T  B  E  S
W  U  A  X  M  B  J  M  V  N  A  I  Q  S  N
F  C  F  Y  S  I  Y  I  Z  M  N  A  G  O  E
A  O  C  Y  T  E  C  I  O  O  S  N  V  L  L
E  O  L  C  E  U  L  R  C  G  G  Y  W  U  E
L  R  K  M  F  H  U  O  O  Y  T  Z  T  V
Y  V  U  C  C  L  E  U  S  S  B  F  I  I
A  C  B  T  A  A  D  V  H  T  C  N  Q  O  T
F  F  Q  N  R  E  S  N  E  D  N  O  C  N  C
Z  E  A  H  O  E  B  U  C  N  G  Y  P  R  E
X  L  B  F  F  U  P  G  I  B  N  E  G  E  J
P  N  A  O  X  I  J  A  G  U  Y  Z  L  L  B
O  Q  A  G  W  B  G  N  O  M  N  Y  O  U  O
```

APERTURE	OBJECTIVELENSES
BINOCULAR	OCULAR
CONDENSER	PLANACHROMATIC
FLUORESCENT	RESOLUTION
MICROSCOPE	

EXERCISE 1.16: FILL-IN-THE-BLANK: THE METRIC SYSTEM AND LABORATORY CALCULATIONS

Instructions: Complete the following chart.

Prefixes for the Multiples and Submultiples of Basic Units

Power of 10	Prefix
_____	kilo
10^1	_____
10^{-1}	_____
_____	centi
10^{-3}	_____
_____	micro
10^{-9}	_____
_____	pico
10^{-15}	_____

Instructions: Answer the following questions.

1. To prepare a 1:10 dilution of a patient sample, combine _____ microliters of sample with 90 microliters of distilled water.

2. Convert 6,234,000 to scientific notation.

   _____

3. Convert 0.0132 to scientific notation.

   _____

4. A pH of 6 is considered neutral. Is this true or false? _____

5. If a standard solution containing 50 mg/mL is diluted 1:5 and 1:10, the final concentrations of the dilutions are _____ and _____, respectively.

The following are the results of control assays for a glucose test on an automated analyzer.

Instructions: Plot the results on the chart below.

Day of the Month	Control Value (mg/dL)
1	93
5	86
8	79
12	81
15	77
19	85
22	90
26	91
29	94

Month <u>August 2018</u>

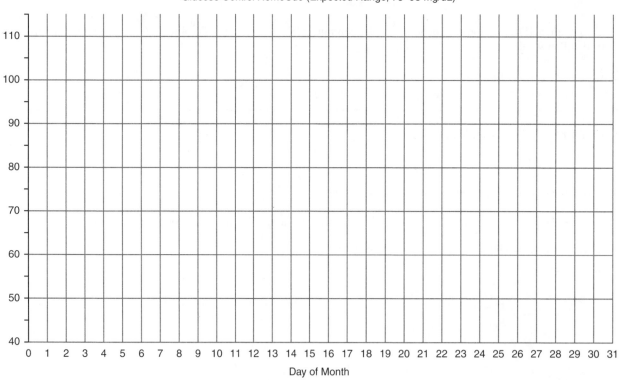

Glucose Control HemoCue (Expected Range, 75–95 mg/dL)

Day of Month

Based on your graph, does the analyzer appear to require maintenance or calibration? Why or why not?

_____

_____

_____

_____

EXERCISE 1.18: QUALITY ASSURANCE CROSSWORD PUZZLE

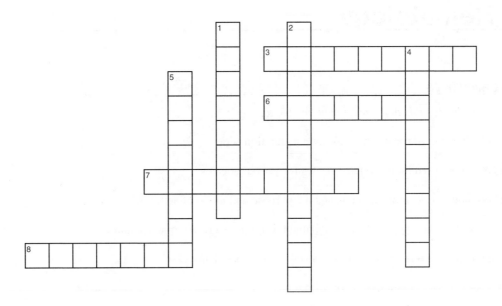

Across

3 Destruction of erythrocytes
6 Presence of fatty material in plasma or serum
7 The magnitude of random errors and the reproducibility of measurements
8 Abnormal yellowish discoloration of skin, mucous membranes, or plasma as a result of increased concentration of bile pigments

Down

1 The closeness with which test results agree with the true quantitative value of the constituent
2 The ability of a method to be accurate and precise
4 Nonbiological solution of an analyte, usually in distilled water, with a known concentration
5 Biological solution of known values used for verification of accuracy and precision of test results

2 Hematology

When you have completed this unit, you should be able to:

1. List the cells in the erythrocyte and leukocyte maturation series.

2. List the commonly used blood collection sites for various species.

3. List the commonly used anticoagulants and the purpose and mode of action for each.

4. List the types of hematology analyzers available for use in veterinary practice and describe their test principles.

5. Perform a complete blood count (CBC) by using an automated analyzer.

6. Define histogram and explain the use of histograms.

7. Perform a packed cell volume test with the microhematocrit method.

8. Calibrate the centrifuge for optimal microhematocrit spin time.

9. Prepare a wedge film to perform a differential leukocyte count.

10. Perform a differential leukocyte count.

11. Identify normal and common abnormal morphology of erythrocytes and leukocytes.

12. Perform a reticulocyte count.

EXERCISE 2.1: HEMATOPOIESIS

Instructions: Answer the following questions.

1. List the cells in the erythrocyte maturation series in order from least to most mature.

_____

_____

2. The primary cytokine responsible for stimulating the production of erythrocytes is

_____.

3. List the cells in the granulocyte maturation series in order from least to most mature.

_____

_____

4. Define leukemoid response.

_____

_____

5. Define pancytopenia.

_____

_____

EXERCISE 2.2: SAMPLE COLLECTION

Instructions: Answer the following questions.

1. List the commonly used blood collection sites for a

   a. Dog _____

   b. Cat _____

   c. Horse _____

   d. Bird _____

2. Explain the difference between serum and plasma.

   _____

   _____

3. The preferred anticoagulant for hematology testing is

   _____.

4. The preferred anticoagulant for coagulation testing is

   _____.

5. The anticoagulant of choice that preserves blood glucose is

   _____.

6. If blood is to be drawn for coagulation and hematology testing, which tube is drawn first?

   _____

Instructions: Complete the following chart.

Cap Color	Additive	Primary Use
7. _____	Sodium citrate	Coagulation studies
Red	Glass: Plastic:	8.
Red/gray or red/black "Tiger top"	Gel separator and clot activator	
Green	9.	10.
11.	EDTA	Hematology
Gray	Potassium oxalate or sodium fluoride	12.

EXERCISE 2.3: LABORATORY EXERCISE: PACKED CELL VOLUME/CENTRIFUGE CALIBRATION

Procedure:

1. Use a stopwatch to verify the centrifuge timer operation. Run several tests at different time intervals, and repeat each at least twice to verify reproducibility.

2. Use a tachometer to check the centrifuge speed if you can view the centrifuge head with the cover in place.

3. Verify the minimum time required to obtain an accurate packed cell volume (PCV).

   The minimum time to achieve optimal packing of the red blood cells (RBCs) should be checked with the following procedure.

   a. Choose two fresh ethylenediaminetetraacetic acid (EDTA)–anticoagulated blood samples. (One sample should have hematocrit [Hct] <50%.)

   b. Fill 10 to 12 microhematocrit tubes for each sample.

   c. Perform duplicate microhematocrit determinations at increasing times, beginning at 2 minutes. Centrifuge times should be increased by 30-second intervals. Record duplicate values at each time interval.

   d. Continue to increase centrifuge time until the value remains the same for two consecutive time intervals.

   e. Centrifuge two more samples for an additional 30 and 60 seconds beyond that interval.

   f. Plot the results on a graph. The plateau point is the first point on the curve after the curve flattens out. This is the optimal spin time.

   g. Repeat the procedure periodically because brushes and motors can become worn out, reducing the speed of the centrifuge.

EXERCISE 2.4: LABORATORY EXERCISE: DETERMINATION OF THE PACKED CELL VOLUME (MICROHEMATOCRIT)

Procedure:

1. Obtain an EDTA-anticoagulated blood sample.

2. Mix the sample by gently inverting it several times.

3. Remove the cap, and tilt the blood tube until the blood is near the mouth of the tube.

4. Hold two capillary tubes together, and insert the tips of the tube into the blood.

5. Allow the tubes to fill about three-quarters full by capillary action.

6. Remove the tubes, and wipe any excess blood off the outside of the tube.

7. Seal the tube ends with clay.

8. Place the tubes in the centrifuge, with the clay plugs facing outward and with the tubes directly opposite each other.

9. Secure the centrifuge lid in place.

10. Set the timer and speed of the centrifuge.

11. Centrifuge for the prescribed time and at the prescribed speed.

12. Allow the centrifuge to come to a complete stop.

13. Determine PCV by using a microhematocrit reader.

14. Alternatively, use a ruler to measure the total height from the top of the clay plug to the top of the plasma column. Make a second measurement from the top of the clay plug to the top of the packed RBC column. Divide the RBC column measurement by the total height to obtain the PCV percentage.

Instructions: Record your results below.

Date _____ Patient name _____ Species _____ Age _____

PCV tube 1 _____ PCV tube 2 _____ Average (PCV1 + PCV2/2) _____

Date _____ Patient name _____ Species _____ Age _____

PCV tube 1 _____ PCV tube 2 _____ Average (PCV1 + PCV2/2) _____

EXERCISE 2.5: INTRODUCTION TO HEMATOLOGY ANALYZERS AND THE COMPLETE BLOOD COUNT

Instructions: Answer the following questions.

1. What information is included in a CBC?

_____

_____

_____

_____

2. Describe the principle of an electrical impedance analyzer.

_____

_____

_____

_____

3. Describe the laser flow cytometry test principles.

_____

_____

_____

_____

4. Describe the principle of quantitative buffy coat analysis.

_____

_____

EXERCISE 2.6: DEFINING KEY TERM

1. Define histogram, and explain the use of histograms.

_____

_____

_____

_____

2. Differentiate between controls and standards.

_____

_____

_____

_____

3. Define the erythrocyte indices.

_____

_____

_____

_____

4. Define buffy coat.

_____

_____

_____

_____

5. Define apoptosis.

_____

_____

_____

_____

Across

1 Cells that have a variable staining pattern; basophilia
2 An RBC with multiple small projections evenly spaced over the cell
3 Group of enzymes with similar catalytic activities but different physical properties
4 The fluid portion of blood after it has clotted; does not contain cells or coagulation proteins.
6 Phagocytic cell derived from the monocyte
9 Another name for a platelet; cytoplasmic fragment of bone marrow megakaryocyte
11 Variation in the size of erythrocytes
13 An immature RBC that contains organelles (ribosomes) that are lost as it matures
14 Erythrocyte fragments formed when the RBC is damaged by intravascular trauma

Down

1 Abnormal shape of erythrocytes
5 A formation of erythrocytes in rows or stacks
7 Increased numbers of leukocytes in the blood
8 Abnormal decrease in neutrophils in a peripheral blood sample
10 Cells with a smaller than normal diameter
12 Round, darkly stained RBCs

EXERCISE 2.8: HEMATOLOGY WORD SEARCH

Instructions: Find the words that are defined by the clues given below. The words may be located horizontally, vertically, or diagonally and may be reversed.

```
M  L  Y  E  T  O  T  A  T  I  E  K  S  R  A
E  E  M  T  A  D  T  M  T  S  A  I  T  N  L
I  O  O  Y  T  E  O  I  N  E  S  T  H  I  M
E  S  N  C  C  E  E  H  A  Y  H  N  S  R  M
R  I  O  O  S  I  S  Y  L  O  M  E  H  M  T
Y  N  C  R  F  I  E  O  U  E  C  M  I  M  A
T  O  Y  C  A  N  Y  E  G  F  S  F  R  N  T
H  P  T  A  K  R  R  A  A  A  A  I  D  M  Z
R  H  E  M  A  C  Y  T  O  M  E  T  E  R  I
O  I  A  K  S  E  T  Y  C  O  P  I  D  A  R
I  L  E  T  G  Z  E  C  I  N  Y  M  H  M  R
D  I  F  F  E  R  E  N  T  I  A  L  O  S  A
E  E  T  Y  C  O  H  T  N  A  C  A  T  A  N
M  I  C  R  O  F  I  L  A  R  I  A  E  L  E
O  I  I  M  L  O  T  I  A  I  O  I  Y  P  R
```

ACANTHOCYTE	EOSINOPHIL	KARYOLYSIS
ADIPOCYTES	ERYTHROID	MACROCYTE
ANTICOAGULANT	HEINZ	MICROFILARIA
DIFFERENTIAL	HEMACYTOMETER	MONOCYTE
DOHLE	HEMOLYSIS	PLASMA

EXERCISE 2.9: LABORATORY EXERCISE: PREPARATION OF THE PERIPHERAL BLOOD SMEAR

Procedure:

1. Thoroughly clean a glass microscope slide with methanol, and polish it dry with lens tissue or other lint-free material.

2. Obtain an EDTA-anticoagulated blood sample.

3. Mix the sample by gently inverting it several times. Remove the cap.

4. Hold two wooden applicator sticks together, and insert them into the tube of blood.

5. Withdraw the sticks from the tube so that 1 drop of blood is between them, *or* remove 1 drop of blood by using a plastic transfer pipette.

6. Place the drop of blood toward one end of the slide.

7. Place a second clean spreader slide in front of the blood drop, and draw the spreader slide into the blood drop at an approximate 30-degree angle.

8. Allow the blood to spread along most of the width of the spreader slide.

9. Push the spreader slide forward in a smooth, rapid motion.

10. Gently wave the slide to air dry it, or place it in a slide dryer.

11. Place the air-dried smear in 95% methanol for 30 to 60 seconds.

12. Stain the slide according to the stain manufacturer's directions.

13. Remove excess stain from the back of the slide, and allow the slide to dry.

EXERCISE 2.10: FILL-IN-THE-BLANK AND SHORT ANSWER: HEMATOLOGY REVIEW

Instructions: Fill in each of the spaces provided with the missing word or words that complete the sentence.

1. An increase in the number of immature neutrophils in blood is called _____.

2. The _____ is a large white blood cell (WBC) with a variably shaped nucleus, diffuse chromatin, and cytoplasmic vacuoles.

3. _____ are the most common leukocytes in the peripheral blood of cats and dogs.

4. RBC fragments that are often seen in disseminated intravascular coagulation are _____.

Instructions: Answer the following questions.

5. What information is included in a differential cell count?

_____

_____

_____

_____

6. Describe the morphologic characteristics for the following WBCs, and note any unique features seen in cells from specific species.

  a. Segmented neutrophil

    _____

    _____

  b. Band neutrophil

    _____

    _____

  c. Lymphocyte

    _____

    _____

  d. Monocyte

    _____

    _____

    _____

    _____

  e. Eosinophil

    _____

    _____

    _____

    _____

  f. Basophil

    _____

    _____

    _____

    _____

7. List the morphologic characteristics of a Howell-Jolly body. When would there be an increase in number?

    _____

    _____

8. List the morphologic characteristics of a Heinz body. When would there be an increase in number?

_____

_____

_____

_____

9. Describe the characteristics of the eosinophilic granules for each species.

   a. Canine

   _____

   b. Feline

   _____

   c. Equine

   _____

   d. Bovine

   _____

EXERCISE 2.11: MATCHING: HEMATOLOGY

Instructions: Match each image to its corresponding cell name.

1.

    a. Basophil

2.

    b. Eosinophil

3.

    c. Monocyte

4.

    d. Neutrophil

5.

    e. Lymphocyte

Instructions: Answer the following questions.

1.

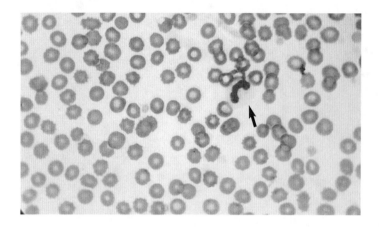

   a. What is the name of the WBC at the pointer?

      —————————————————————

   b. Describe the characteristics of this cell.

      ———

      ———

2.

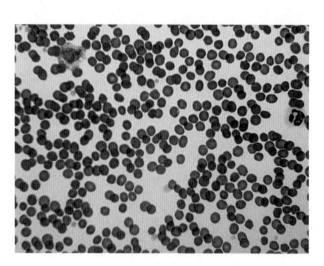

   a. What is the name of the WBC in the upper left corner?

      —————————————————————

   b. Describe the characteristics of this cell.

      ———

      ———

3.

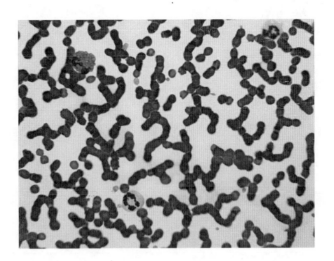

This is a blood smear from a horse.

    a. Name the two WBCs on this blood smear.

    _____

    b. Describe the RBC morphology.

    _____

    _____

4.

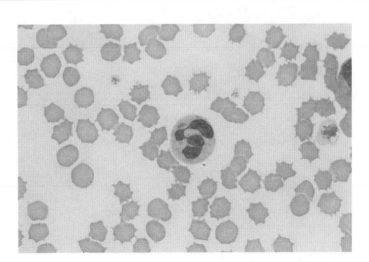

    a. Name the WBC.

    _____

    b. Describe the characteristics of this cell.

    _____

    _____

5.

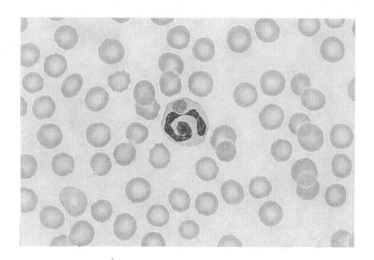

   a. Name the WBC.

   _____

   b. Describe the characteristics of this cell.

   _____

   _____

6.

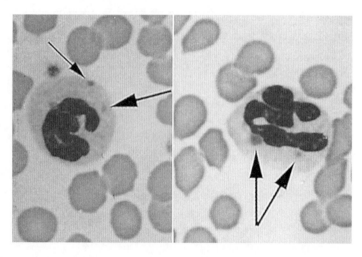

This is a blood smear from a cat.

   a. Name the cells on this slide.

   _____

   b. Describe the characteristics of this cell.

   _____

   _____

7.

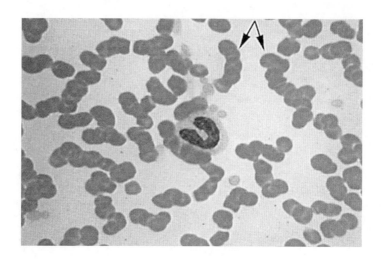

a. Name the WBC.

_____

b. Describe the RBC morphology.

_____

_____

8.

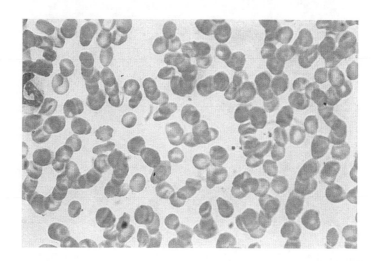

Describe the RBC morphology.

_____

_____

9.

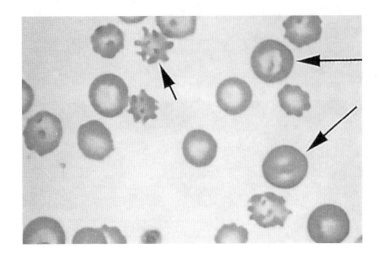

    a. Name the cells at the long arrows.

    _____

    b. Name the cell at the short arrow.

    _____

10.

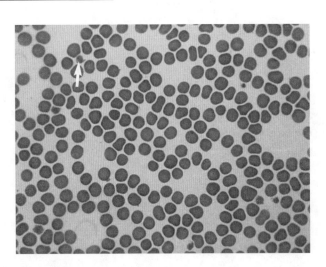

    a. What is the arrow pointing at?

    _____

    b. From what precursor does this arise?

    _____

    c. Describe the RBC morphology on this blood smear.

    _____

    _____

11.

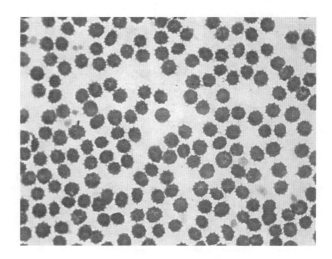

   a. What is occurring on this blood smear with respect to RBC morphology?

     _____

   b. Describe the characteristics of these cells.

     _____

     _____

12.

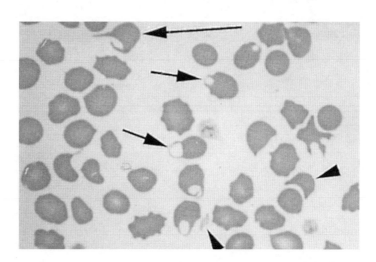

   a. Name the RBC at the long arrow.

     _____

   b. Describe the characteristics of this cell.

     _____

     _____

13.

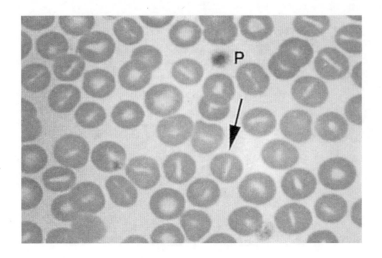

a. Name the RBC at the pointer.

_____

14.

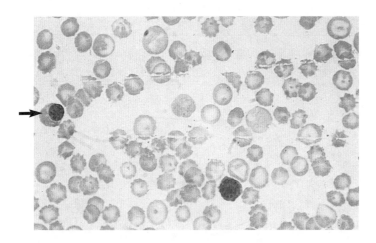

a. What is the name of the cell at the pointer?

_____

b. Is this cell mature or immature?

_____

15.

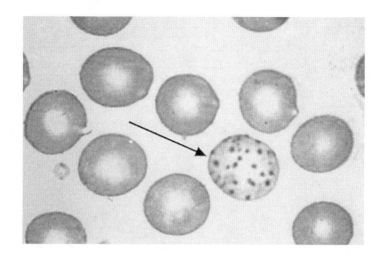

a. Name the RBC at the pointer.

_____

b. What type of toxicity is this characteristic of?

_____

16.

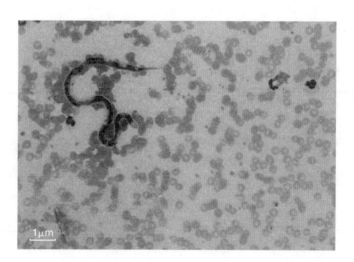

a. What is the name of this blood parasite seen in this blood smear?

_____

17.

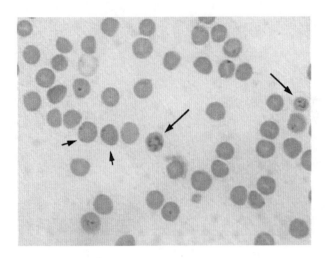

    a. What is the name of the cell at the long arrows (new methylene blue [NMB] stain)?

    _____

    b. Is this cell mature or immature?

    _____

18.

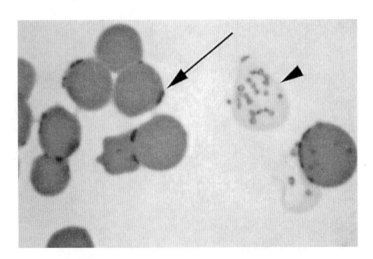

    a. This is a blood smear from a cat. What is the name of the organism on the cell at the pointer?

    _____

    b. Describe the characteristics of this cell.

    _____

    _____

19.

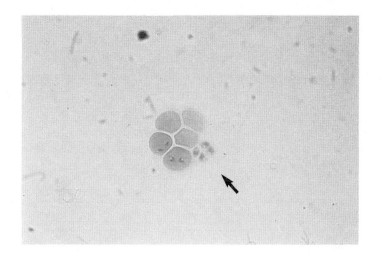

    a. This is a blood smear from a cow. What is the name of the cell at the pointer?

        _____

    b. Describe the characteristics of the intracellular organism.

        _____

        _____

20.

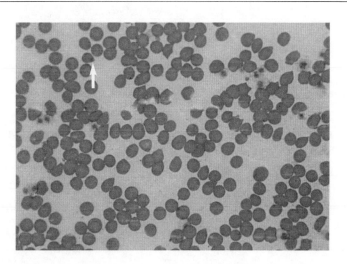

    a. What is the name of the RBC at the arrowhead?

        _____

    b. Describe the characteristics of this cell.

        _____

        _____

    c. Which stain should be used to identify this cell?

        _____

21.

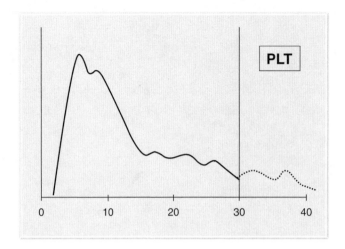

What is indicated by this histogram?

_____

_____

22.

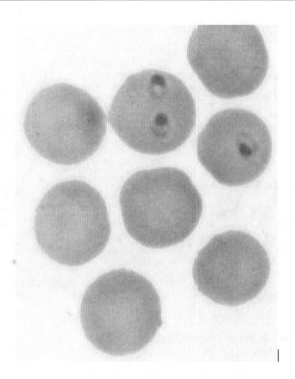

Name the organism present in these RBCs.

23.

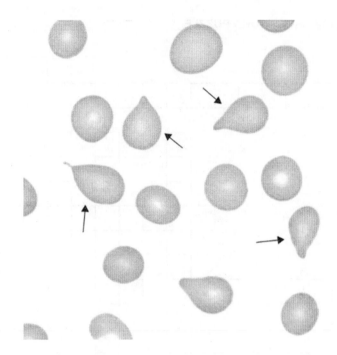

Describe the cells in this image, and explain how to verify that they are not an artifact.

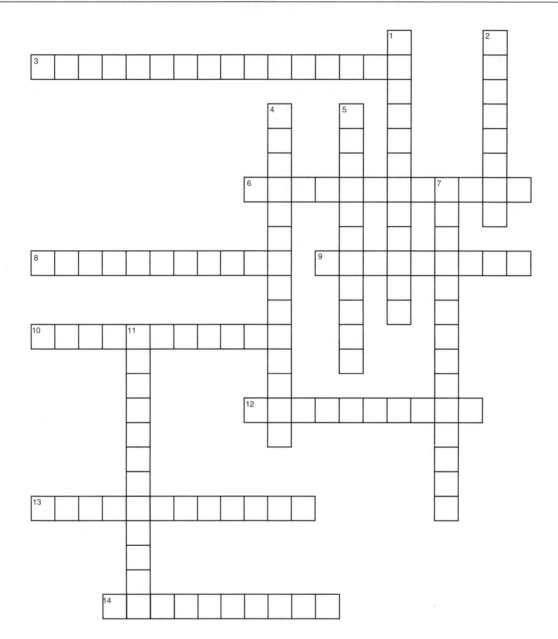

Across

3 Decrease in circulating platelets
6 Production of leukocytes
8 An erythrocyte with spiny projections of different lengths distributed irregularly over the cell; spur cell
9 An erythrocyte with many small projections evenly spaced over the cell
10 Erythrocyte with a linear area of central pallor
12 Leukocyte of avian, reptile, and some fish species containing prominent eosinophilic granules
13 Cells that stain with their characteristic color
14 An abnormally shaped erythrocyte that appears to have horns

Down

1 Decreased numbers of all blood cells and platelets in peripheral blood or bone marrow sample
2 Neoplastic cells in blood or bone marrow
4 Denotes a neutrophil with more than five nuclear lobes
5 RBCs with decreased staining intensity from decrease in hemoglobin concentration
7 Production of erythrocytes
11 Leukocyte group that has no visible cytoplasmic granules

EXERCISE 2.14: LABORATORY EXERCISE: COUNTING RETICULOCYTES

Procedure:

1. Filter a few drops of reticulocyte stain (NMB or brilliant cresyl blue) by passing it through a piece of filter paper, coffee filter, or lint-free tissue.

2. Obtain an EDTA-anticoagulated blood sample from a dog and a cat.

3. Place a few drops of each blood sample in a separate labeled tube.

4. Add an equal volume of the filtered reticulocyte stain.

5. Allow the tubes to stand undisturbed at room temperature for 15 minutes.

6. Clean and thoroughly dry two microscope slides.

7. Label each slide with the patient identification (ID).

8. Withdraw a large drop of the mixture in each tube, and make a thick blood film by using the wedge film technique. Allow the film to dry.

9. Examine each slide with the oil immersion objective.

10. Count 1000 erythrocytes, and record the number of reticulocytes in them.

11. Calculate the reticulocyte percentage.

$$\frac{\# \ of \ reticulocytes}{1000} \times 100 = \% \ reticulocytes$$

12.

    a. Calculate the absolute value of reticulocytes by multiplying the total RBC count, if available, *or*

    b. Calculate the corrected reticulocyte count by using the equation:

        i. Canine : % reticulocytes $\dfrac{PCV\%}{45\%} = corrected \ reticulocyte \ \%$

        ii. Feline : % reticulocytes $\dfrac{PCV\%}{35\%} = corrected \ reticulocyte \ \%$

Record your results.

Patient name _____ Species _____ Date _____

Total # of reticulocytes counted per 1000 RBCs _____ Reticulocyte % _____

Reticulocyte absolute value _____ Corrected reticulocyte % _____

Patient name _____ Species _____ Date _____

Total # of reticulocytes counted per 1000 RBCs _____ Reticulocyte % _____

Reticulocyte absolute value _____ Corrected reticulocyte % _____

Patient name _____ Species _____ Date _____

Total # of reticulocytes counted per 1000 RBCs _____ Reticulocyte % _____

Reticulocyte absolute value _____ Corrected reticulocyte % _____

EXERCISE 2.14 HEMATOLOGY REVIEW QUESTIONS

Instructions: Answer the following questions.

1. Name the two morphologic forms of reticulocytes seen in samples from feline patients.

   _____

   _____

2. Describe the characteristics of the two morphologic forms of reticulocytes seen in samples from feline patients.

   _____

   _____

3. Which form is counted to determine the reticulocyte count in the cat?

   _____

   _____

EXERCISE 2.15: HEMATOLOGY WORD SEARCH

Instructions: Find the words that are defined by the clues given below. The words may be located horizontally, vertically, or diagonally and may be reversed.

```
O  N  R  N  H  E  M  E  E  T  N  T  D  S  D  N
E  O  I  E  O  O  F  E  E  S  O  N  M  A  S  A
T  I  R  C  O  T  A  M  E  H  O  R  C  I  M  E
Y  T  O  E  O  G  I  T  Y  L  A  R  X  N  O  N
C  A  H  L  B  R  N  S  T  L  Y  E  I  E  L  C
O  N  G  P  I  O  B  E  I  O  H  B  M  P  Y  P
Y  I  N  M  E  H  O  C  R  O  F  Y  O  C  O
R  T  R  A  B  Y  P  Y  R  L  I  K  L  H  I  O
A  U  M  D  N  O  T  O  G  B  N  E  E  P  D  R
K  L  O  O  S  E  Y  O  R  O  P  G  Y  M  U  A
A  G  R  A  I  R  M  I  S  T  H  N  C  Y  O  P
G  G  B  K  A  E  N  I  O  L  U  E  E  L  A  L
E  A  A  K  H  O  S  C  A  P  I  E  I  D  M  A
M  I  T  C  I  T  Y  C  O  M  R  O  N  T  L  O
P  S  S  M  K  T  E  O  R  T  U  A  I  N  I  M
M  R  A  A  E  P  S  I  I  Y  B  E  E  I  Y  N
```

AGGLUTINATION	FIBRIN	MEGAKARYOCYTE
ANEMIA	HEMOGLOBIN	MICROHEMATOCRIT
BAND	KARYORRHEXIS	NEUTROPHIL
BASOPHIL	LEPTOCYTE	NORMOCYTIC
DACRYOCYTE	LYMPHOPENIA	PYKNOSIS

Hematology Report Form

Patient name: _____ Date: _____

Species: _____ Breed: _____ Age: _____ Gender: _____

Collection date/time: _____

WBC count	
RBC count	
Platelet count	
PCV (mHCT)	
TP (Total protein)	
Hemoglobin	
MCV	
MCH	
MCHC	

WBC differential:

	Relative	Absolute
Segmented neutrophil		
Non-segmented (band) neutrophil		
Lymphocyte		
Monocyte		
Eosinophil		
Basophil		

Platelet estimation:

_____

_____

_____

RBC morphology:

_____

_____

_____

Comments:

_____

_____

_____

Hematology Report Form

Patient name: _____ Date: _____

Species: _____ Breed: _____ Age: _____ Gender: _____

Collection date/time: _____

WBC count	
RBC count	
Platelet count	
PCV (mHCT)	
TP (Total protein)	
Hemoglobin	
MCV	
MCH	
MCHC	

WBC differential: Relative   Absolute

	Relative	Absolute
Segmented neutrophil		
Non-segmented (band) neutrophil		
Lymphocyte		
Monocyte		
Eosinophil		
Basophil		

Platelet estimation:

_____

_____

_____

RBC morphology:

_____

_____

_____

Comments:

_____

_____

_____

Hematology Report Form

Patient name: _____ Date: _____

Species: _____ Breed: _____ Age: _____ Gender: _____

Collection date/time: _____

WBC count	
RBC count	
Platelet count	
PCV (mHCT)	
TP (Total protein)	
Hemoglobin	
MCV	
MCH	
MCHC	

WBC differential: Relative   Absolute

	Relative	Absolute
Segmented neutrophil		
Non-segmented (band) neutrophil		
Lymphocyte		
Monocyte		
Eosinophil		
Basophil		

Platelet estimation:

_____

_____

_____

RBC morphology:

_____

_____

_____

Comments:

_____

_____

_____

3 Hemostasis

LEARNING OBJECTIVES

When you have completed this unit, you should be able to:

1. Explain the role of platelets in blood coagulation.

2. Describe the events that occur during blood coagulation.

3. Discuss proper sample collection for hemostatic tests.

4. Describe methods to estimate platelet numbers.

5. List the tests used to evaluate the chemical phases of blood coagulation.

6. Perform a manual fibrinogen estimate.

7. Perform the buccal mucosa bleeding time test.

8. Perform the activated clotting time (ACT) test.

EXERCISE 3.1: FILL-IN-THE-BLANK AND SHORT ANSWER: HEMOSTASIS REVIEW

Instructions: Answer the following questions and fill in each of the spaces provided with the missing word or words that complete the sentence.

1. The _____ phase is initiated when a blood vessel is ruptured or torn.

2. _____ serves to stabilize the platelet plug.

3. _____ are membrane-bound cytoplasmic fragments released from platelets, leukocytes, and endothelial cells on which coagulation complexes can form.

4. When platelets are activated, _____ is exposed on the outer surface of the membrane.

5. Samples for coagulation testing are mixed with sodium citrate anticoagulant in a ratio of _____.

6. The _____ test can evaluate every clinically significant clotting factor except Factor VII.

7. The ACT test uses a tube containing _____ or _____.

8. The most common inherited coagulation disorder of domestic animals is _____.

9. _____ is a coagulation disorder characterized by the depletion of platelets and coagulation factors.

10. _____ is the most common inherited coagulation factor deficiency in dogs and is caused by Factor _____ deficiency.

11. List at least five clinical signs associated with defects or deficiencies of platelets.

_____

_____

_____

_____

_____

_____

12. Which coagulation factors require vitamin K for synthesis and activation?

_____

13. On a differential blood smear, _____ platelets per oil-immersion field are seen in normal patients.

14. _____ represents the mathematic average of the size of the individual platelets counted by the analyzer.

15. Another term for *platelets* is _____.

16. Describe two methods for estimating platelet numbers.

_____

_____

_____

_____

_____

_____

EXERCISE 3.2: DEFINING KEY TERMS

Instructions: Define each term in your own words.

1. D-Dimers

_____

2. Megakaryocyte

_____

3. Thrombocytopenia

_____

4. Prothrombin time

_____

5. Petechia

_____

EXERCISE 3.3: WORD SEARCH: HEMOSTASIS

Instructions: Find the words that are defined by the clues given below. The words may be located horizontally, vertically, or diagonally and may be reversed.

```
C E T Q R U L Q V H L J R V R K M O K Q
N G N J T Y G F C Z V Y B V F E I K E A
M Q Y I H B J G K E A V J L L Y C C U I
Y H P A R G O T S A L E O B M O R H T N
V Y Z W O E R L J A T Z A O T K O A I E
D I C D M H S Y L I K L N H B Y P S R P
I E E R B W Q L R C U V R E S G A Y C O
Z P V R I I D C Y G Y O I V T L R E T T
X M L V N D O N A D M F F P P H T I E Y
O O O C I B R O A B I O E I G A I D L C
K H T M M C K O R C T N Z H K C T E O
E C E O V R S C R Z B Q A O P X L B T B
A R R E W Y N W V M E T H V B E M A M
S H F P Y T N I R B I F L U P E S B L O
T H Y P O C O A G U L A B L E S T A P R
A H M S G O C O N Q L U D Z I F O T S H
G A I H T A P O B M O R H T L W P H E T
I S G E J H T P H C W X Z Q M M N C P Y
D D L D Y Y F I B R O M E T E R V O V Q
U R N H Y D L T A O N W B W R J X O V H
```

ACT	FIBROMETER	PHOSPHATIDYLSERINE	THROMBOCYTOPENIA
BMBT	HYPERCOAGULABLE	PIVKA	THROMBOCYTOSIS
D-DIMERS	HYPOCOAGULABLE	PLATELETCRIT	THROMBOELASTOGRAPHY
DIC	MICROPARTICLES	THROMBIN	THROMBOPATHIA
FIBRIN	MONOVETTE	THROMBOCRIT	VONWILLEBRAND

51

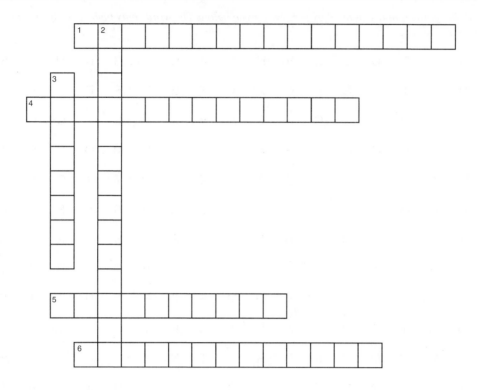

Across

1 Decrease in circulating platelets
4 Production of platelets
5 An instrument used in hemostatic evaluation of samples
6 Bone marrow cell from which blood platelets arise

Down

2 Characterized by abnormally decreased coagulability
3 Formed from prothrombin, calcium, and thromboplastin in plasma during the clotting process

EXERCISE 3.5: LABORATORY EXERCISE: BUCCAL MUCOSA BLEEDING TIME TEST

Procedure:

1. Anesthetize the patient, and place the patient in lateral recumbency.

2. Fold back the lip, and secure it with gauze.

3. Place the lancet device against the mucosal surface at the level of the premolars.

4. Depress the trigger on the device without pressing against the mucosa, and simultaneously start the timer.

5. After 5 seconds, wick the blood away from the incision site with filter paper. Do not touch the actual incision.

6. Continue removal of the blood drop every 5 seconds until the filter paper comes up clean.

7. Record the time.

Record your results:

Date _____

Patient ID _____ Species_____ Gender_____ Age _____

Bleeding time _____

Date_____

Patient ID _____ Species _____ Gender _____ Age _____

Bleeding time _____ Date _____

Date _____

Patient ID _____ Species _____ Gender _____ Age _____

Bleeding time _____

EXERCISE 3.6: LABORATORY EXERCISE: MANUAL FIBRINOGEN ESTIMATE

Procedure:

1. Fill two hematocrit tubes, and centrifuge them as for a packed cell volume (PCV).

2. Determine the total solids (TS) on one tube with a refractometer.

3. Incubate the second tube at 58° C for 3 minutes.

4. Recentrifuge the second tube.

5. Determine the total solids on the second tube with a refractometer.

6. Multiply the total solids in grams per deciliter (g/dL) by 1000 to obtain the concentration in milligrams per deciliter (mg/dL).

7. Calculate the fibrinogen estimate with the following equation (with all values in milligrams per deciliter):

$$\text{TS mg/dL}_{(nonincubated)} - \text{TS mg/dL}_{(incubated)} = \text{Estimated fibrinogen mg/dL}$$

Record your results:

Date _____

Patient ID _____ Species _____ Gender _____ Age _____

TS in tube 1 _____ TS in tube 2 _____

Fibrinogen estimate _____

Date _____

Patient ID _____ Species _____ Gender _____ Age _____

TS in tube 1 _____ TS in tube 2 _____

Fibrinogen estimate _____

Date _____

Patient ID _____ Species _____ Gender _____ Age _____

TS in tube 1 _____ TS in tube 2 _____

Fibrinogen estimate _____

EXERCISE 3.7: LABORATORY EXERCISE: ACTIVATED CLOTTING TIME

Procedure:

1. Prewarm the ACT tube in a 37° C heat block or water bath for 20 minutes.

2. Perform venipuncture using a sterile syringe with no additive.

3. Begin timing when blood first enters the syringe.

4. Place 2 mL of blood into the prewarmed ACT tube.

5. Cap and gently invert the tube one time.

6. Place filled tube in a heat block or water bath.

7. Beginning at 60 seconds:

    a. Remove the tube from the heat block or water bath, and tilt it to look for evidence of clotting.

    b. Return the tube to the heat block or water bath.

    c. Repeat a and b above every five seconds until a visible clot is evident.

Record your results:

Date _____

Patient ID _____ Species _____ Gender _____ Age _____

ACT _____ _____

Date _____

Patient ID _____ Species _____ Gender _____ Age _____

ACT _____ _____

Date _____

Patient ID _____ Species _____ Gender _____ Age _____

ACT _____ _____

Coagulation Profile

Patient name: _____ Date: _____

Species: _____ Breed: _____ Age: _____ Gender: _____

Test	
Platelets $\times 10^3/\mu L$	
Mean platelet volume (fl)	
Thrombin time (seconds)	
Prothrombin time (seconds)	
PTT (seconds)	
APTT (seconds)	
Fibrinogen (mg/dL)	
Bleeding time (minutes)	
ACT (seconds)	

Coagulation Profile

Patient name: _____ Date: _____

Species: _____ Breed: _____ Age: _____ Gender: _____

Test	
Platelets $\times 10^3/\mu L$	
Mean platelet volume (fl)	
Thrombin time (seconds)	
Prothrombin time (seconds)	
PTT (seconds)	
APTT (seconds)	
Fibrinogen (mg/dL)	
Bleeding time (minutes)	
ACT (seconds)	

Coagulation Profile

Patient name: _____ Date: _____

Species: _____ Breed: _____ Age: _____ Gender: _____

Test	
Platelets $\times 10^3/\mu L$	
Mean platelet volume (fl)	
Thrombin time (seconds)	
Prothrombin time (seconds)	
PTT (seconds)	
APTT (seconds)	
Fibrinogen (mg/dL)	
Bleeding time (minutes)	
ACT (seconds)	

4 Immunology

LEARNING OBJECTIVES

When you have completed this unit, you should be able to:

1. Differentiate between innate immunity and adaptive immunity.

2. Differentiate between humoral immunity and cell-mediated immunity.

3. List the five classes of immunoglobulins and state the structure and primary role of each.

4. Define immunologic tolerance.

5. Describe the various populations of T lymphocytes and B lymphocytes and explain the role of each in the immune system.

6. Differentiate between passive immunity and active immunity.

7. Discuss sensitivity and specificity as they relate to immunologic test kits.

8. List the types of diagnostic test kits that are available for the in-house veterinary practice laboratory.

9. Describe the principle of enzyme-linked immunosorbent assay (ELISA) testing.

10. Describe the principle of latex agglutination testing.

11. Perform blood typing and crossmatching.

12. Describe common immune system disorders.

EXERCISE 4.1: REVIEW QUESTIONS

Instructions: Answer the following questions.

1. List the components that comprise the innate immune system.

_____

_____

_____

_____

_____

_____

2. Define antigen.

_____

_____

3. Describe the events that comprise the inflammatory response.

_____

_____

_____

_____

_____

_____

_____

_____

_____

_____

_____

4. List the signs of inflammation.

_____

_____

_____

_____

5. List the cells in the maturation series of lymphocytes.

_____

_____

_____

_____

6. Define immunologic tolerance.

_____

_____

7. Define cytokine.

_____

_____

8. State the general principle of ELISA tests.

_____

_____

_____

_____

_____

_____

_____

_____

_____

_____

_____

9. Activation of the complement system can lead to _____, _____, or _____.

10. The primary function of B lymphocytes is production of _____ as part of the humoral immune system.

11. The most abundant circulating immunoglobulin is _____.

12. _____ reactions occur when antigens bind with antibodies and form an insoluble complex.

13. _____ refers to the ability of the test to correctly identify all animals that test truly positive in a given reaction procedure.

14. The _____method is the most common type of immunoassay used in veterinary practice laboratories.

15. Atopy and anaphylaxis are type _____ hypersensitivity disorders.

16. Glomerulonephritis is an example of type _____ hypersensitivity.

17. In dogs, which blood group elicits the greatest antigen response and causes the most serious transfusion reactions if mismatched blood is administered? _____

18. The vast majority of cats in the United States have blood group _____.

19. In cats, the most serious transfusion reactions occur with administration of type _____ blood to type _____ cats.

20. Blood typing of dogs and cats can be performed in the veterinary practice laboratory with either the _____ or the _____ method.

21. Define humoral immunity.

_____

_____

22. Define antibody titer.

_____

_____

23. Name two immunologic tests that are based on the principles of cell-mediated immunity.

_____

_____

_____

24. Describe the mechanism involved in type I hypersensitivity reactions.

_____

_____

_____

_____

_____

_____

_____

25. Name at least two antibody-mediated type II hypersensitivity reactions.

_____

_____

EXERCISE 4.2: IMMUNOLOGY CROSSWORD PUZZLE

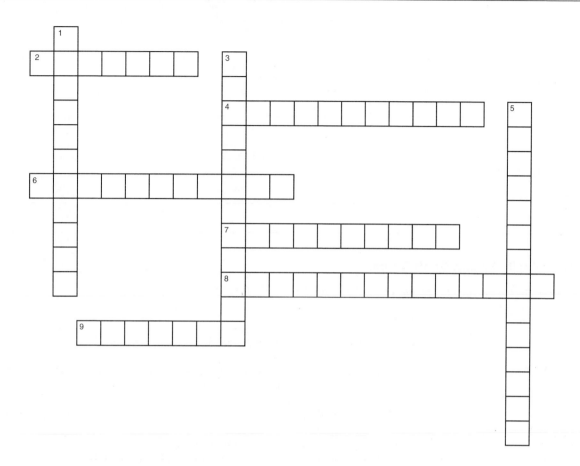

Across

2 Enzyme-linked immunosorbent assay
4 A measure of the numbers of false positives produced with the given reaction procedure
6 Refers to the ability of the test to correctly identify all animals that are truly positive for a given reaction procedure
7 Edema of the dermis and subcutaneous tissues
8 An antibody
9 Any substance capable of generating a response from the immune system

Down

1 Soluble proteins secreted by cells to mediate immune responses that elicit other cellular reactions
3 Refers to binding of complement to antigen
5 A naturally occurring antibody produced by an individual that reacts with alloantigens of another individual of the same species

EXERCISE 4.3: KEY TERMS

1. Define avidity.

_____

_____

2. Define chemiluminescence.

_____

_____

3. Define alloantibodies.

_____

_____

4. Define urticaria.

_____

_____

5. Define angioedema.

_____

_____

EXERCISE 4.4: IMMUNOLOGY MATCHING

Instructions: Match the immunoglobulin (Ig) class with each of the functions.

Immunoglobulin Class

1. _____ IgG

2. _____ IgM

3. _____ IgE

4. _____ IgA

5. _____ IgD

Function

a. B-lymphocyte surface antigen receptor in some species

b. Neutralization of microbes and toxins; fetal and neonatal immunity by passive transfer across placenta and in colostrum

c. Mucosal immunity; protection of respiratory, intestinal, and urogenital tracts

d. Immediate hypersensitivity reactions, such as allergies and anaphylactic shock; coating of helminth parasites for destruction by eosinophils

e. Activation of complement

EXERCISE 4.5: WORD SEARCH: IMMUNOLOGY

Instructions: Find the words that are defined by the clues given below. The words may be located horizontally, vertically, or diagonally and may be reversed.

```
Y  Q  C  B  B  T  J  G  S  H  G  A  H  M  P  Y  Y  Y  U  P
Q  H  A  R  T  I  T  E  R  F  U  U  X  P  A  K  T  N  D  C
R  Y  P  J  O  Y  T  X  D  T  C  I  K  S  B  F  I  P  Y  O
N  F  R  A  Z  S  T  J  O  B  R  G  S  E  S  R  V  P  K  L
J  D  I  P  R  O  S  I  Y  U  P  A  T  G  R  U  I  S  O  P
O  R  Q  S  O  G  M  M  X  N  O  L  L  F  A  Y  T  L  C  Z
S  D  D  M  Q  M  O  I  A  N  U  C  K  I  Z  Z  I  A  K  O
X  W  J  L  U  K  B  T  U  T  Z  G  C  W  E  Y  S  E  I  E
E  L  U  N  G  A  B  M  A  W  C  T  M  B  V  D  N  H  X  V
Z  Q  E  H  R  J  M  T  F  M  L  H  R  J  F  E  E  W  O  A
O  E  A  F  I  I  C  Q  F  A  O  D  I  Q  H  X  S  J  K  C
U  F  J  C  O  U  B  A  Q  A  D  R  A  N  O  V  R  D  U  C
J  S  B  I  U  M  B  B  I  S  E  Z  H  P  G  O  E  I  O  I
T  N  D  O  Y  W  S  L  A  R  R  L  F  C  Z  H  P  N  O  N
P  A  V  X  P  D  C  O  L  J  A  L  S  N  O  Y  Y  S  B  A
R  E  N  I  M  A  T  S  I  H  E  C  N  X  P  N  H  J  Y  T
I  M  M  U  N  O  D  I  F  F  U  S  I  O  N  L  U  Q  T  I
D  Z  S  N  E  D  D  D  A  U  T  P  T  T  Z  D  A  M  D  O
P  T  Y  H  R  H  K  Z  S  H  Q  A  A  N  R  E  B  U  M  N
H  S  E  H  L  O  Y  E  G  A  I  I  J  D  V  U  O  T  B  I
```

ATOPY	IMMUNODIFFUSION
AUTOIMMUNE	RADIOIMMUNOASSAY
CROSSMATCHING	TITER
HISTAMINE	URTICARIA
HYPERSENSITIVITY	VACCINATION
IMMUNOCHROMATOGRAPHY	WHEALS

EXERCISE 4.6: FILL-IN-THE-BLANK: IMMUNOASSAYS

Instructions: Complete the following chart for the immunoassays available in your laboratory.

Name of Test	Manufacturer	Principle (if ELISA, state format—e.g., microwell, filter)	Use

Procedure:

1. Obtain whole blood samples (in ethylenediaminetetraacetic acid [EDTA] anticoagulant) from the donor and the recipient.

   ■ Samples may also be obtained from stored whole blood or packed red blood cells (pRBCs).

2. Centrifuge the EDTA tubes at 1000 g for 10 minutes. Remove the plasma, and place it in labeled tubes.

3. Place 3 to 5 drops of the pRBCs from each EDTA tube into the labeled conical centrifuge tubes.

4. Add 5 to 10 mL of saline to the pRBCs.

5. Centrifuge the tubes with pRBCs for 2 to 5 minutes.

6. Pour off the supernatant, and discard it.

7. Resuspend the pRBCs in saline, and centrifuge them.

   a. Repeat steps 6 and 7 one to three times until the supernatant is clear.

8. Add a few drops of saline to resuspend the pRBCs.

9. **Major crossmatch:** Label a plain tube with the donor name and "major."

   a. Add 2 drops of the recipient plasma and 2 drops of donor cell suspension.

10. **Minor crossmatch:** Label a tube with the donor number and "minor."

    a. Add 2 drops of the donor plasma and 2 drops of the recipient cell suspension.

11. **Controls:** Label two control tubes.

    a. Add 2 drops of donor plasma and 2 drops of donor RBCs to the first tube.

    b. Add 2 drops of recipient plasma and 2 drops of recipient RBCs to the second tube.

12. Incubate all four tubes at 37° C (98.6° F) for 15 to 30 minutes.

    a. Room temperature incubation is sometimes performed and generally yields accurate results.

13. Centrifuge all four tubes for 5 minutes.

14. Examine all four tubes macroscopically for evidence of hemolysis or agglutination.

15. Grade any agglutination reactions, and examine the samples microscopically.

16. Positive reactions in the donor control tubes indicate unsuitable donors.

Grade	Description
0	No evidence of agglutination or hemolysis
1	Many small agglutinates and some free cells
2	Large agglutinates and smaller clumps of cells
3	Many large agglutinates
4	Solid aggregate of cells

Blood Typing and Crossmatching Report

Patient name: _____Date: _____

Species: _____ Breed: _____ Age: _____ Gender: _____

Blood type test method: _____

Blood type result: _____

Crossmatching: _____

Donor ID: _____

Crossmatch method: _____

Crossmatch result: _____

Blood Typing and Crossmatching Report

Patient name: _____Date: _____

Species: _____ Breed: _____ Age: _____ Gender: _____

Blood type test method: _____

Blood type result: _____

Crossmatching: _____

Donor ID: _____

Crossmatch method: _____

Crossmatch result: _____

Blood Typing and Crossmatching Report

Patient name: _____Date: _____

Species: _____ Breed: _____ Age: _____ Gender: _____

Blood type test method: _____

Blood type result: _____

Crossmatching: _____

Donor ID: _____

Crossmatch method: _____

Crossmatch result: _____

Blood Typing and Crossmatching Report

Patient name: _____Date: _____

Species: _____ Breed: _____ Age: _____ Gender: _____

Blood type test method: _____

Blood type result: _____

Crossmatching: _____

Donor ID: _____

Crossmatch method: _____

Crossmatch result: _____

5 Urinalysis

LEARNING OBJECTIVES

When you have completed this unit, you should be able to:

1. List the methods used to obtain samples for urinalysis.

2. Describe proper sample handling of urine samples.

3. Prepare urine for microscopic examination.

4. Perform physical and chemical evaluation of urine.

5. Perform microscopic examination of urine.

6. List crystals that may be encountered in urine sediment.

7. Describe the formation of casts and explain their significance in a urine sample.

8. List and describe parasites that may be encountered in urine sediment.

EXERCISE 5.1: FILL-IN-THE-BLANK

Instructions: Fill in each of the spaces provided with the missing word or words that complete the sentence.

1. Pigments that give color to urine are called _____.

2. _____ is defined as an increase in the frequency of urination.

3. A decrease in the volume of urine produced is called _____.

4. A _____ urine sample is collected while the animal urinates.

5. _____ is a method of collecting urine for culture and sensitivity and can be used if a _____ cannot be performed.

6. _____ occurs when the specific gravity of urine approaches that of the glomerular filtrate (1.008–1.012).

7. _____ properties of urine include volume, color, odor, turbidity, and specific gravity.

8. An increase in the total volume of urine produced is called _____.

9. _____ properties of urine are usually evaluated with the use of reagent strips or reagent tablets.

10. A _____ crystal is commonly seen in alkaline to slightly acidic urine; sometimes referred to as a triple phosphate crystal.

11. _____ crystals are commonly seen in the urine of rabbits and horses.

12. The presence of calculi (stones) in the urinary tract is called _____.

13. _____ crystals are formed in acidic and neutral urine; commonly resemble the back of an envelope.

14. _____ are formed in the lumen of the distal and collecting tubules of the kidney, where the concentration and acidity of urine are greatest.

15. The three types of _____ cells found in urinary sediment are squamous, transitional, and renal.

EXERCISE 5.2: URINALYSIS CROSSWORD PUZZLE

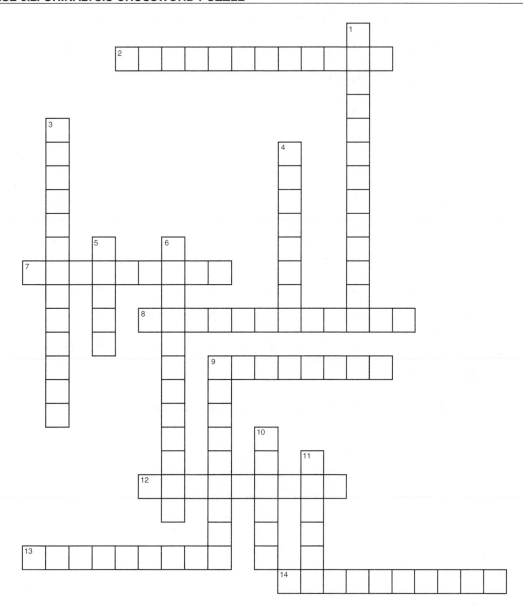

Across

2 Cells smaller than a WBC; may be smooth, biconcave disk shape
7 Term used for presence of RBCs in urine
8 Urine specific gravity approaches glomerular filtrate
9 Crystals referred to as triple phosphate crystals
12 Type of water used to calibrate a refractometer
13 Protein found in muscle; urine is very dark brown
14 Cells larger than RBCs and smaller than renal epithelial cells

Down

1 Instrument used to determine specific gravity
3 Sterile collection of urine; can be used for culture and sensitivity
4 pH above 7.0
5 Formed in the lumen of the distal and collecting tubules of the kidney
6 Presence of crystals in urine
9 Stain used for observing cells in urine sediment
10 Physical properties of urine include color, odor, turbidity, specific gravity, and _____
11 _____ bodies are formed during incomplete catabolism of fatty acids

69

Instructions: Find the words that are defined by the clues given below. The words may be located horizontally, vertically, or diagonally and may be reversed.

```
B  M  W  H  Y  C  Q  G  L  W  A  T  C  C  S
I  W  E  X  V  M  S  V  U  I  G  K  A  I  B
L  M  D  G  Z  O  K  T  R  G  A  Q  S  Z  M
I  A  O  I  U  K  B  U  R  L  M  E  T  Y  N
R  I  Z  B  A  F  T  E  O  U  T  U  O  L  E
U  R  S  E  B  A  I  M  W  N  V  G  Y  J  W
B  U  Y  J  M  K  X  R  E  M  L  I  W  V  F
I  S  R  E  F  R  A  C  T  O  M  E  T  E  R
N  O  H  C  S  M  O  U  B  N  Z  H  E  E  V
U  C  Z  H  Q  T  P  I  O  G  E  W  R  H  O
R  U  Q  J  S  L  N  L  D  N  Y  C  F  G  J
I  L  L  Y  Y  U  O  L  I  G  U  R  I  A  L
A  G  C  R  R  U  H  R  K  O  X  G  Y  Y  D
O  C  S  I  S  A  I  H  T  I  L  O  R  U  G
V  S  A  I  T  F  L  T  Y  G  N  H  J  M  V
```

BILIRUBINURIA	MYOGLOBINURIA
CAST	OLIGURIA
CENTRIFUGE	REFRACTOMETER
CYSTOCENTESIS	STRUVITE
GLUCOSURIA	UROLITHIASIS
HEMATURIA	

EXERCISE 5.4: LABORATORY EXERCISE: URINE SAMPLE COLLECTION BY CATHETERIZATION

Procedure:

1. Choose the proper type and size urinary catheter for a dog.

   a. For female dogs:

      i. Clip the area free of hair, and prepare the site aseptically.

      ii. Use a sterile vaginal speculum to visualize the urethra.

   b. For male dogs:

      i. Extrude the penis aseptically, and prepare the area without touching the prepuce.

2. Lubricate the distal end of the catheter, and handle the catheter aseptically.

3. Introduce and pass the catheter into the bladder, and avoid contamination.

4. Empty the bladder with a syringe or attach a collection system to the catheter.

EXERCISE 5.5: LABORATORY EXERCISE: URINE SAMPLE COLLECTION BY CYSTOCENTESIS

Procedure:

1. Select a 22- or 20-gauge needle by 1 inch or 1½ inches and a 10-mL syringe.

2. Place the animal in lateral recumbency, ventral recumbency, or in the standing position.

3. Palpate and immobilize the bladder.

4. Insert the needle into the caudal abdomen in the dorsocaudal direction.

   a. For male dogs, insert the needle caudal to the umbilicus and to the side of the sheath.

   b. For female dogs and for cats, insert the needle on the ventral midline caudal to the umbilicus.

5. Gently aspirate urine into the syringe, and properly label it with the patient's information.

EXERCISE 5.6 URINALYSIS REVIEW QUESTIONS

Instructions: Answer the following questions.

1. Describe four methods of urine collection. Include the technique used for each, and describe which method is best used for culture and sensitivity.

   _____

   _____

   _____

   _____

   _____

   _____

2. List the physical properties evaluated in a urinalysis.

_____

_____

_____

3. Why is horse urine normally cloudy?

_____

_____

_____

4. Why is it important to use a fresh urine sample when performing a complete urinalysis?

_____

_____

_____

5. What should be performed to a refractometer before each use?

_____

_____

_____

6. Define specific gravity.

_____

_____

_____

7. List the factors that may cause a decrease as well as an increase in the urine pH.

_____

_____

_____

_____

_____

_____

_____

_____

8. When preparing urine sediment for microscopic examination, what is the maximum amount of urine (in milliliters) that should be placed into a labeled conical centrifuge tube? How long and at what speed should a urine sample be centrifuged?

_____

_____

_____

9. Briefly describe the procedure for urine sediment examination.

_____

_____

_____

_____

_____

_____

_____

_____

_____

10. When examining urine sediment under a microscope, what objective should be used?

_____

_____

_____

_____

_____

_____

11. List and describe the crystals that may be seen in acidic and alkaline urine.

_____

_____

_____

_____

_____

_____

12. Describe the characteristics of an erythrocyte in fresh urine sediment when examining it under a microscope.

_____

_____

_____

_____

_____

_____

_____

_____

13. Describe the characteristics of a leukocyte in fresh urine when examining it under a microscope.

_____

_____

_____

14. List the five main types of casts seen in urine sediment, and provide a brief description of each.

_____

_____

_____

_____

_____

_____

15. List the three types of epithelial cells found in urine sediment from the largest to the smallest.

_____

_____

_____

16. Describe renal threshold.

_____

_____

17. List six changes to urine as it sits at room temperature for more than 1 hour.

_____

_____

_____

_____

_____

_____

18. Normal urine output for both canines and felines is _____ mL/lb in 24 hours.

19. Glucose in the urine is called _____ or _____.

20. List the six causes of ketonuria.

_____

_____

_____

_____

_____

_____

21. Define hematuria.

_____

_____

22. Define hemoglobinuria.

_____

_____

23. How can hemoglobinuria be differentiated from hematuria?

_____

_____

24. Squamous epithelial cells originate in the _____ _____, vagina, _____, or _____.

25. In concentrated urine, erythrocytes will _____.

26. Define ghost cells.

_____

_____

27. From where do transitional epithelial cells originate?

_____

_____

28. How are granular casts formed?

_____

_____

29. Name the type of urine crystal often referred to as _triple phosphate_.

_____

30. Name the type of urinary crystal most commonly associated with ethylene glycol poisoning.

_____

_____

EXERCISE 5.6: LABORATORY EXERCISE: PHYSICAL AND CHEMICAL EVALUATIONS OF URINE

Procedure:

1. Obtain a 10-mL urine sample. (Smaller volumes can be used, but test results may be inaccurate.)

2. Pour the sample into a clean, dry, clear container (test tube or specimen cup).

3. Evaluate the sample's color.

4. Evaluate the sample's turbidity.

5. Evaluate the specimen's odor.

6. Perform specific gravity evaluation with a refractometer.

7. Note the condition and expiration date of urine dipstick test strips.

8. Immerse the dipstick in the urine sample. Note the time.

9. Remove the dipstick, and place it on a paper towel.

10. Tilt the dipstick on its long edge to wick away excess urine from the dipstick.

11. Evaluate the color changes at the prescribed times as stated on the dipstick package.

12. Record the results on the urinalysis report form.

EXERCISE 5.7: LABORATORY EXERCISE: MICROSCOPIC EVALUATION OF URINE

Procedure:

1. Pour approximately 10 mL (5 mL minimum) of the urine sample into a labeled conical centrifuge tube.

2. Centrifuge the sample for 3 to 6 minutes at 1000 to 2000 rpm.

3. Pour off the supernatant, leaving approximately 0.5 to 1 mL in the tube.

4. Resuspend the sediment by flicking the tube with your fingers or by gently mixing the sediment and supernatant with a pipette.

5. Transfer 1 drop of resuspended sediment near the end of a microscope slide with a transfer pipette, and place a coverslip over it.

6. *Optional:* Add 1 drop of Sedi-Stain or new methylene blue (NMB) stain to 1 drop of urine sediment on the other end of the microscope slide, and place a coverslip over it.

7. Subdue the light of the microscope by partially closing the iris diaphragm.

8. Scan the entire unstained slide for the presence of large formed elements, such as casts and clusters of cells.

9. Examine the entire specimen under the coverslip with the high-power (40×) objective to identify and quantify formed elements. Use the stained sediment, as needed, to confirm identification of the formed element.

10. Examine a minimum of 10 microscopic fields with the high-power lens.

11. Record the results. Report cells and bacteria in numbers/high-power field (HPF) and casts in numbers/low-power field (LPF). The report can list either the average number seen in 10 microscope fields or a range representing the lowest and the highest numbers of each element seen in 10 microscopic fields.

EXERCISE 5.8: PHOTO QUIZ: URINALYSIS

Instructions: Answer the following questions.

1.

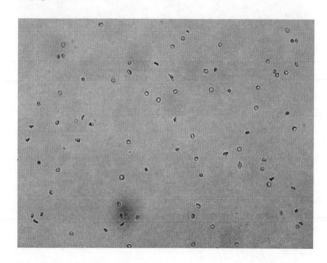

What cells are observed in this urine sediment slide?

_____

_____

2.

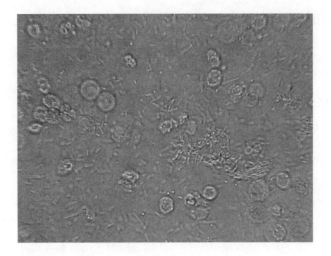

What cells are observed in this urine sediment slide?

_____

_____

3.

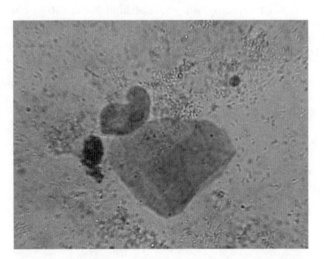

a. What is the name of the large cell?

_____

b. Describe the characteristics of this cell, and explain from where it is derived.

_____

_____

4.

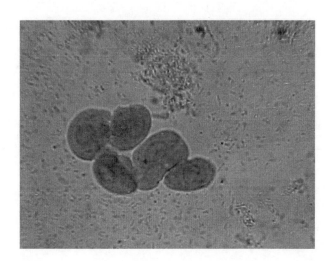

    a. What are the clusters of cells?

_____

_____

    b. Describe the characteristics of this cell type, and explain from where it is derived.

_____

_____

5.

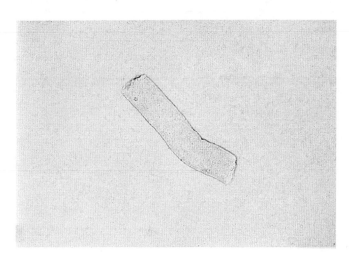

    a. What is the name of the structure present?

_____

    b. Describe the characteristics of this formed element.

_____

_____

6.

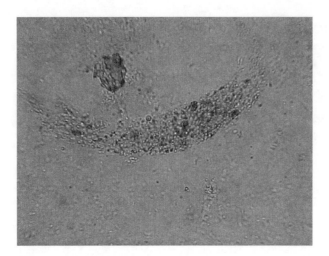

a. What is the name of this cast?

_____

b. Describe the characteristics of this cast.

_____

_____

7.

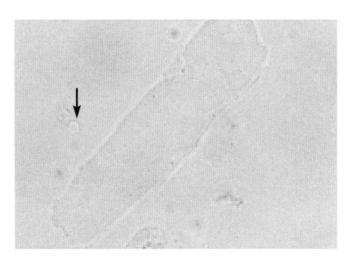

a. What is the name of this cast?

_____

b. Describe the characteristics of this cast.

_____

_____

8.

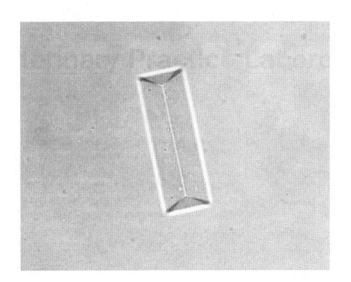

    a. Name the crystal.

_____

    b. In what pH is this crystal found?

_____

    c. Describe the shape of the crystal.

_____

_____

9.

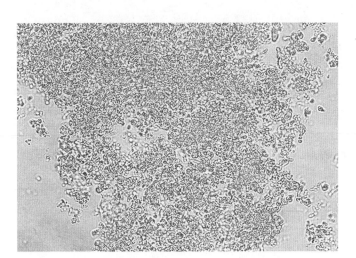

    a. Name the crystal on this slide.

_____

    b. In what pH is this crystal found?

_____

_____

10.

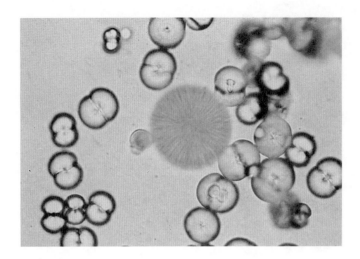

a. Name the crystal on this slide.

_____

b. In what two species are these normally seen?

_____

_____

11.

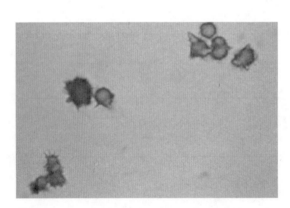

a. Name the crystal on this slide.

_____

b. In what pH is this crystal found?

_____

c. Describe the shape of this crystal.

_____

_____

12.

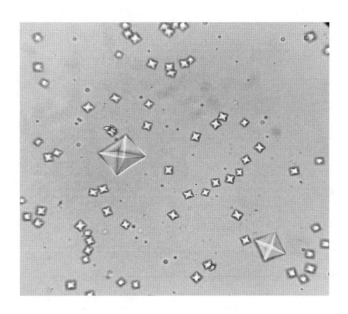

a. Name the crystal on this slide.

_____

b. In what pH is this crystal found?

_____

c. Describe the shape of this crystal.

_____

_____

13.

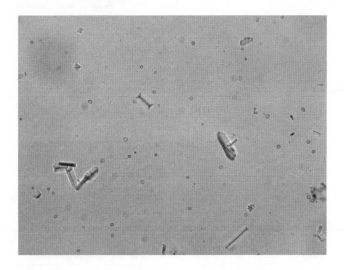

Name the cells and crystals observed in this urine sediment slide.

_____

14.

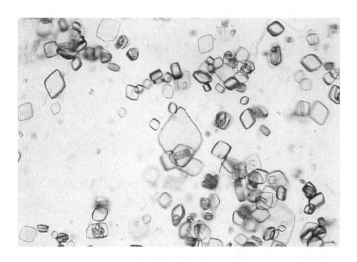

   a. Name the crystals observed in this urine sediment slide.

_____

   b. Describe the shape of this crystal.

_____

_____

15.

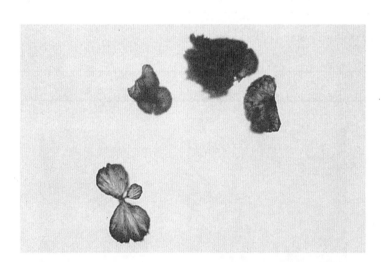

   a. Name these crystals.

_____

   b. In what pH is this crystal found?

_____

_____

   c. Describe the characteristics of this crystal.

_____

_____

16.

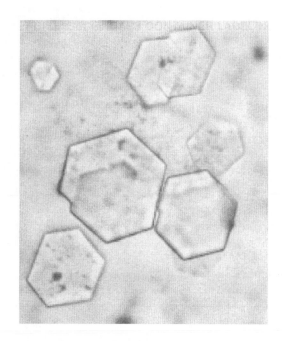

    a. Name the crystal on this slide.

_____

    b. In what pH is this crystal found?

_____

    c. Describe the shape of this crystal.

_____

_____

17.

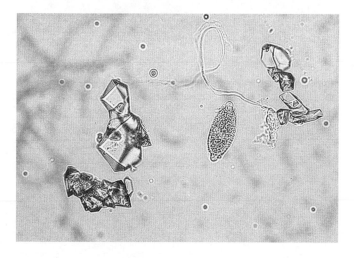

Name the parasite ova in this urine sediment slide.

_____

18.

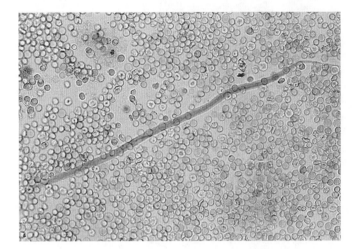

Name the parasite seen in this urine sediment slide.

_____

19.

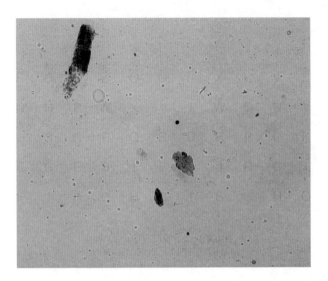

Name the structures or cells observed in this urine sediment.

_____

20.

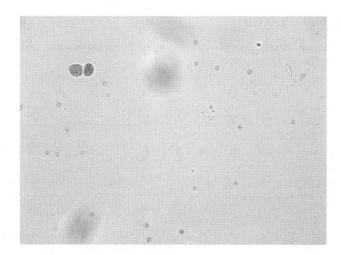

Name the cells in the upper left side of this urine sediment.

_____

Instructions: Find the words that are defined by the clues given below. The words may be located horizontally, vertically, or diagonally and may be reversed.

```
T  L  Y  X  A  W  Y  S  S  C  Q  A  L  S  B
M  A  U  M  E  X  K  I  F  R  Q  U  O  E  J
O  I  I  F  V  E  R  S  A  Z  C  V  X  N  Q
E  L  S  U  L  U  R  E  M  O  L  G  G  O  I
R  E  T  W  O  P  D  T  B  P  Y  C  N  T  E
Y  H  U  U  N  C  O  N  J  U  G  A  T  E  D
T  T  R  F  I  L  Y  E  B  Q  I  M  D  K  N
H  I  B  R  R  E  E  C  U  N  W  N  R  I  S
R  P  I  L  E  U  K  O  C  Y  T  E  A  E  H
0  E  D  U  H  C  B  T  L  E  N  T  D  Q  O
C  Q  I  X  M  I  B  S  B  A  S  I  Y  C  T
Y  Y  T  O  K  N  K  Y  L  I  M  P  M  O  L
T  A  Y  T  J  E  K  C  D  E  I  I  B  G  G
E  O  X  A  L  A  T  E  N  I  S  O  R  Y  T
P  N  F  O  J  N  S  T  U  H  V  H  C  V  F
```

CYSTOCENTESIS	RENAL
EPITHELIAL	SEDIMENT
ERYTHROCYTE	SEDISTAIN
GLOMERULUS	TURBIDITY
KETONES	TYROSINE
LEUCINE	UNCONJUGATED
LEUKOCYTE	WAXY
OXALATE	

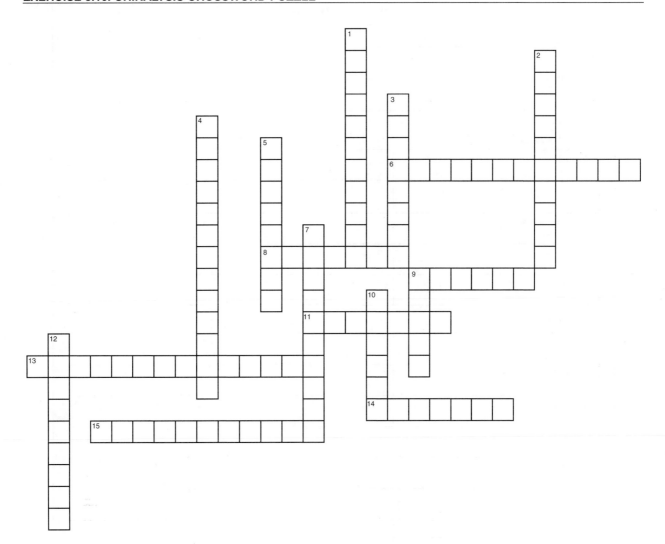

Across

6 _____bilirubin does not pass through the glomerulus into the renal filtrate and is not water soluble
8 Calcium _____ crystals are seen in urine of animals poisoned with ethylene glycol
9 Calcium carbonate crystals are commonly seen in the horse and _____
11 Animals with liver disease may have these crystals; wheel or pincushion shaped
13 A result of intravascular hemolysis
14 Conditions that lead to crystal formation may also cause formation of urinary _____
15 Seen in urine sediment of intact male animals

Down

1 Often seen with traumatic catheterization or bladder expression
2 Type of bilirubin found in urine
3 Crystal that resembles a coffin lid
4 Seen in horses with exertional rhabdomyolysis
5 Largest of the epithelial cells
7 _____ plica is a bladder worm of dogs and cats
9 Smallest epithelial cell observed in urine
10 pH below 7.0
12 Occurs in animals with diabetes mellitus

Urinalysis Report Form

Patient name: _____ Date: _____

Species: _____ Breed: _____ Age: _____ Gender: _____

Collection date/time: _____ Method of collection: _____

Physical properties

Volume:	
Color:	
Appearance/turbidity:	
Odor:	
Specific gravity:	

Chemical properties

pH:	
Protein:	
Glucose:	
Ketones:	
Urobilinogen:	
Bilirubin:	
Hemoglobin:	
Blood:	

Urine sediment

RBC (HPF):	
WBC (HPF):	
Epithelial cells (HPF): specify type	
Bacteria (HPF):	
Crystals (HPF): specify type	

Comments:	

Urinalysis Report Form

Patient name: _____ Date: _____

Species: _____ Breed: _____ Age: _____ Gender: _____

Collection date/time: _____ Method of collection: _____

Physical properties

Volume:	
Color:	
Appearance/turbidity:	
Odor:	
Specific gravity:	

Chemical properties

pH:	
Protein:	
Glucose:	
Ketones:	
Urobilinogen:	
Bilirubin:	
Hemoglobin:	
Blood:	

Urine sediment

RBC (HPF):	
WBC (HPF):	
Epithelial cells (HPF): specify type	
Bacteria (HPF):	
Crystals (HPF): specify type	

Comments:	

Urinalysis Report Form

Patient name: _____ Date: _____

Species: _____ Breed: _____ Age: _____ Gender: _____

Collection date/time: _____ Method of collection: _____

Physical properties

Volume:	
Color:	
Appearance/turbidity:	
Odor:	
Specific gravity:	

Chemical properties

pH:	
Protein:	
Glucose:	
Ketones:	
Urobilinogen:	
Bilirubin:	
Hemoglobin:	
Blood:	

Urine sediment

RBC (HPF):	
WBC (HPF):	
Epithelial cells (HPF): specify type	
Bacteria (HPF):	
Crystals (HPF): specify type	

Comments:	

6 Clinical Chemistry

LEARNING OBJECTIVES

When you have completed this unit, you should be able to:

1. Prepare serum and plasma samples for chemistry analyses.

2. Describe the effects of sample compromise on test results.

3. Describe the principles of common analyzer types.

4. List the chemical tests used for the evaluation of liver, kidney, and pancreatic functions.

5. List the major electrolyte assays performed with in-house analyzers.

6. Perform clinical chemistry analyses.

EXERCISE 6.1: FILL-IN-THE-BLANK: REVIEW

Instructions: Fill in each of the spaces provided with the missing word or words that complete the sentence.

1. Chemical measurements should be completed within _____ after blood collection.

2. A blood sample from an animal that has not eaten for 12 hours is a _____ sample.

3. _____ is the fluid portion of whole blood in which the cells are suspended.

4. A chemical analyzer that uses a prism to select a specific wavelength of light is a _____, and an analyzer that uses a filter to select the wavelength is a _____.

5. Increases in _____ bilirubin indicate problems with uptake (hepatic damage).

6. Increases in _____ bilirubin indicate bile duct obstruction.

7. Cholesterol assay is sometimes used as a screening test for _____.

8. The common enzyme tests of liver function performed in small animal veterinary practice are _____.

9. Isoenzymes of _____ are present in osteoblasts, chondroblasts, and the cells of the hepatobiliary system in the liver.

10. The primary serum chemistry tests for kidney function are _____ and _____.

11. In most mammalian species, _____ is converted to allantoin before being excreted in the urine.

12. Uric acid is the major end product of nitrogen metabolism in _____ species and is also seen in _____ dogs.

13. The _____ test evaluates glomerular function by using test substances eliminated by both glomerular filtration and renal secretion.

14. A type of test that describes the excretion of specific electrolytes relative to the glomerular filtration rate is

_____.

15. Tests of the endocrine functions of the pancreas include _____, _____, and _____.

16. Increased fructosamine indicates a persistent hyperglycemia of _____ in dogs and cats.

17. Increased _____ indicates a persistent hyperglycemia of 3 to 4 months in dogs and 2 to 3 months in cats.

18. The ketone produced in greatest abundance in ketoacidotic patients is _____.

19. The kidneys play a major role in regulating the concentration of _____ by actively secreting or resorbing it from the filtrate in response to the blood pH.

20. Increased levels of _____ indicate hypoperfusion or hypoxia.

EXERCISE 6.2: CLINICAL CHEMISTRY CROSSWORD PUZZLE

Across

6 Equipment designed to measure the amount of light transmitted through a solution

Down

1 Represents the irreversible reaction of glucose bound to protein
2 Increased retention of urea in the blood
3 An insoluble molecule derived from the breakdown of hemoglobin
4 The major binding and transport protein in the blood; responsible for maintaining osmotic pressure of plasma
5 Plasma from which fibrinogen has been removed
7 The fluid portion of whole blood in which the cells are suspended

Instructions: Answer the following questions.

1. List at least three causes of hemolysis in samples.

   _____

   _____

   _____

2. State the calculation used for a one-point calibration assay.

   _____

   _____

3. List at least two possible causes of hyperproteinemia and hypoproteinemia.

   _____

   _____

4. List at least two conditions associated with hypernatremia and hyponatremia.

   _____

   _____

5. List at least two conditions associated with hyperkalemia and hypokalemia.

   _____

   _____

6. Define azotemia, and explain why dehydration is usually accompanied by azotemia.

   _____

   _____

   _____

   _____

7. List the tests commonly performed to evaluate the acinar functions of the pancreas.

   _____

   _____

8. Define acute-phase proteins, and name the two most commonly evaluated acute-phase proteins in small animals.

   _____

   _____

9. Define cholestasis.

_____

_____

10. Describe the general principle of photometry.

_____

_____

_____

_____

_____

_____

EXERCISE 6.4: CLINICAL CHEMISTRY WORD SEARCH

Instructions: Find the words that are defined by the clues given below. The words may be located horizontally, vertically, or diagonally and may be reversed.

```
L  R  O  N  A  E  N  H  P  E  H  N  J  M  Y  H  R
I  L  E  D  I  I  S  L  R  Y  K  A  V  V  I  E  Q
P  A  U  F  L  B  A  A  P  X  U  U  C  G  T  M  C
A  T  U  U  L  S  U  E  L  N  U  F  Y  E  D  A  O
S  Z  S  I  M  E  R  R  D  Y  H  U  M  S  S  T  R
E  N  O  A  S  C  C  I  I  E  M  O  K  U  I  O  T
I  A  U  T  A  H  C  T  C  L  T  A  I  R  S  C  I
H  G  C  P  E  E  B  N  O  O  I  B  I  E  Y  H  S
W  H  N  I  A  M  A  O  H  M  S  B  F  T  L  E  O
N  I  Y  M  N  D  I  P  M  B  E  F  E  C  O  Z  L
A  H  E  M  E  A  O  A  Q  E  Y  T  B  I  M  I  L
N  E  F  P  Z  R  R  Z  L  M  U  R  E  S  E  A  M
B  M  M  Y  T  A  C  I  D  O  S  I  S  R  H  B  H
F  I  Z  C  S  I  S  O  L  A  K  L  A  P  B  Y  B
C  T  E  L  I  P  E  M  I  A  N  I  M  U  B  L  A
O  P  E  A  D  A  J  A  V  I  K  G  K  X  U  R  L
S  H  Y  P  E  R  G  L  Y  C  E  M  I  A  F  E  C
```

ACIDOSIS	BILIRUBIN	ICTERUS	PLASMA
ACINAR	CORTISOL	IMPEDANCE	REFLECTOMETER
ALBUMIN	HEMATOCHEZIA	INSULIN	SERUM
ALKALOSIS	HEMOLYSIS	JAUNDICE	SPECTROPHOTOMETER
AMYLASE	HYPERCAPNIA	LIPASE	
AZOTEMIA	HYPERGLYCEMIA	LIPEMIA	

EXERCISE 6.5: LABORATORY EXERCISE: PLASMA SAMPLE PREPARATION

Procedure:

1. Collect a blood sample in a container with the appropriate anticoagulant.

2. Mix the blood-filled container with a gentle rocking motion 12 times.

3. Make sure the container is covered to prevent evaporation during centrifugation.

4. Centrifuge (within 1 hour of collection) at 2000 to 3000 rpm for 10 minutes.

5. With a capillary pipette, carefully remove the fluid plasma layer from the bottom layer of cells.

6. Transfer the plasma to a container labeled with the date, time of collection, patient's name, and case or clinic number.

7. Process immediately, or refrigerate or freeze, as appropriate.

EXERCISE 6.6: LABORATORY EXERCISE: SERUM SAMPLE PREPARATION

Procedure:

1. Collect a whole blood sample in a container that contains no anticoagulant.

2. Allow the blood to clot in its original container at room temperature for 20 to 30 minutes.

3. Gently separate the clot from the container by running a wooden applicator stick around the wall of the container between the clot and the wall.

4. Cover the sample and centrifuge at 2000 to 3000 rpm for 10 minutes.

5. With a capillary pipette, remove the serum from the clot.

6. Transfer the serum to a container labeled with the date, time of collection, patient's name, and clinic or case number.

7. Refrigerate or freeze the sample, as appropriate

EXERCISE 6.7: HEMATOLOGY ANALYZERS

Instructions: Complete the following data for all the analyzers in your laboratory.

Name of analyzer _____

Technology (circle):

    spectrophotometer   photometer   reflectometer   ion selective electrode   electrochemical
                                                                       (ISE) analyzer

Test menu (circle):   single tests only   profiles only   profiles or single tests

List tests that the analyzer can perform.

_____

_____

_____

Are preassayed controls available for the analyzer? _____

How often are controls run and recorded? _____

Are control results graphed? _____

What types of specimens can be used? (circle)

    serum   plasma   whole blood   other (specify) _____

How are test results obtained? (circle)

    printout   displayed   integrated directly   other (specify) _____
                                               into patient record

List the steps, in order, for performing a test with this analyzer.

_____

_____

_____

_____

_____

Name of analyzer _____

Technology (circle):

    spectrophotometer   photometer   reflectometer   ISE analyzer   electrochemical

Test menu (circle):   single tests only   profiles only   profiles or single tests

List tests that the analyzer can perform.

_____

_____

_____

Are preassayed controls available for the analyzer? _____

How often are controls run and recorded? _____

Are control results graphed? _____

What types of specimens can be used? (circle)

    serum   plasma   whole blood   other (specify) _____

How are test results obtained? (circle)

    printout   displayed   integrated directly   other (specify) _____
                                               into patient record

List the steps, in order, for performing a test with this analyzer.

_____

_____

_____

_____

_____

Name of analyzer _____

Technology (circle):

    spectrophotometer   photometer   reflectometer   ISE analyzer   electrochemical

Test menu (circle):   single tests only   profiles only   profiles or single tests

List tests that the analyzer can perform.

_____

_____

_____

Are preassayed controls available for the analyzer? _____

How often are controls run and recorded? _____

Are control results graphed? _____

What types of specimens can be used? (circle)

    serum   plasma   whole blood   other (specify) _____

How are test results obtained? (circle)

    printout   displayed   integrated directly   other (specify) _____
                                  into patient record

List the steps, in order, for performing a test with this analyzer.

_____

_____

_____

_____

_____

_____

Name of analyzer _____

Technology (circle):

    spectrophotometer   photometer   reflectometer   ISE analyzer   electrochemical

Test menu (circle):   single tests only   profiles only   profiles or single tests

List tests that the analyzer can perform.

_____

_____

_____

Are preassayed controls available for the analyzer? _____

How often are controls run and recorded? _____

Are control results graphed? _____

What types of specimens can be used? (circle)

    serum   plasma   whole blood   other (specify) _____

How are test results obtained? (circle)

    printout   displayed   integrated directly   other (specify) _____
                                        into patient record

List the steps, in order, for performing a test with this analyzer.

_____

_____

_____

_____

_____

Clinical Chemistry Profile

Date _____ Patient ID _____ Species _____

Breed _____ Gender _____ Age _____

Sample type (circle):   venous   arterial   capillary

Time collected _____

Analyzer used _____	Units	Result
Albumin		
ALT		
AST		
ALP		
Amylase		
Bile acids: fasting		
Bile acids: 2-hour postprandial		
Bilirubin, total		
Bilirubin, direct		
Calcium		
Cholesterol		
Creatine kinase		
Creatinine		
Glucose		
Lipase		
Protein, total serum		
SDH		
Urea nitrogen		
Analyzer used _____		
Bicarbonate (mEq/L)		
Chloride (mEq/L)		
Magnesium (mg/dL)		
Phosphorus (mg/dL)		
Potassium (mEq/L)		
Sodium (mEq/L)		
Analyzer used _____		
pH		
PCO_2		
TO_2		
HCO_3		
TCO_2		

Clinical Chemistry Profile

Date _____ Patient ID _____ Species _____

Breed _____ Gender _____ Age _____

Sample type (circle):   venous   arterial   capillary

Time collected _____

Analyzer used _____	Units	Result
Albumin		
ALT		
AST		
ALP		
Amylase		
Bile acids: fasting		
Bile acids: 2-hour postprandial		
Bilirubin, total		
Bilirubin, direct		
Calcium		
Cholesterol		
Creatine kinase		
Creatinine		
Glucose		
Lipase		
Protein, total serum		
SDH		
Urea nitrogen		
Analyzer used _____		
Bicarbonate (mEq/L)		
Chloride (mEq/L)		
Magnesium (mg/dL)		
Phosphorus (mg/dL)		
Potassium (mEq/L)		
Sodium (mEq/L)		
Analyzer used _____		
pH		
PCO_2		
TO_2		
HCO_3		
TCO_2		

Clinical Chemistry Profile

Date _____ Patient ID _____ Species _____

Breed _____ Gender _____ Age _____

Sample type (circle):   venous   arterial   capillary

Time collected _____

Analyzer used _____	Units	Result
Albumin		
ALT		
AST		
ALP		
Amylase		
Bile acids: fasting		
Bile acids: 2-hour postprandial		
Bilirubin, total		
Bilirubin, direct		
Calcium		
Cholesterol		
Creatine kinase		
Creatinine		
Glucose		
Lipase		
Protein, total serum		
SDH		
Urea nitrogen		
Analyzer used _____		
Bicarbonate (mEq/L)		
Chloride (mEq/L)		
Magnesium (mg/dL)		
Phosphorus (mg/dL)		
Potassium (mEq/L)		
Sodium (mEq/L)		
Analyzer used _____		
pH		
PCO_2		
TO_2		
HCO_3		
TCO_2		

Clinical Chemistry Profile

Date _____ Patient ID _____ Species _____

Breed _____ Gender _____ Age _____

Sample type (circle):   venous   arterial   capillary

Time collected _____

Analyzer used _____	Units	Result
Albumin		
ALT		
AST		
ALP		
Amylase		
Bile acids: fasting		
Bile acids: 2-hour postprandial		
Bilirubin, total		
Bilirubin, direct		
Calcium		
Cholesterol		
Creatine kinase		
Creatinine		
Glucose		
Lipase		
Protein, total serum		
SDH		
Urea nitrogen		
Analyzer Used _____		
Bicarbonate (mEq/L)		
Chloride (mEq/L)		
Magnesium (mg/dL)		
Phosphorus (mg/dL)		
Potassium (mEq/L)		
Sodium (mEq/L)		
Analyzer used _____		
pH		
PCO_2		
TO_2		
HCO_3		
TCO_2		

7 Microbiology

LEARNING OBJECTIVES

When you have completed this unit, you should be able to:

1. Describe the characteristic shapes and arrangements of bacteria.

2. List the commonly used culture media and state the characteristics of the media.

3. Perform the Gram staining procedure.

4. Describe commonly used staining procedures for microbiology samples.

5. Inoculate culture media.

6. Perform antibiotic sensitivity testing.

7. Perform dermatophyte testing.

8. Perform catalase testing.

EXERCISE 7.1: DEFINING KEY TERMS

Instructions: Define each term in your own words.

1. Selective medium

_____

_____

_____

2. Differential medium

_____

_____

_____

3. Enrichment medium

_____

_____

_____

4. Transport medium

_____

_____

_____

Instructions: Answer the following questions.

1. Why are samples to be Gram stained heat fixed before staining?

_____

_____

2. List three methods of sample collection for microbiology.

_____

_____

_____

3. What reagent should be used to prepare a solid tissue sample for fungal testing?

_____

_____

4. Name two types of dermatophyte test media.

_____

_____

5. Name the broth media that is commonly used for urine cultures.

_____

6. The catalase test is used to help identify gram-_____ _____ and small gram-_____

_____.

7. The reagent used for the catalase test is _____ _____.

8. The majority of clinically significant bacterial species requires a pH in the range of _____.

9. _____ bacteria prefer reduced oxygen tension, and _____ bacteria require high levels of carbon dioxide.

10. Most pathogenic bacteria thrive at temperatures of _____.

11. Bacterial shapes are described as _____, _____, _____, and _____.

12. Fungal organisms consist largely of webs of slender tubes called _____.

106

13. Partial hemolysis that creates a narrow band of greenish or slimy discoloration around the bacterial colony is referred to as _____.

14. The _____ test is used to aid bacterial classification when gram-variable results are obtained.

15. _____ stain is primarily used to detect the organisms of *Mycobacterium* and *Nocardia* species.

16. Hairs infected with some species of _____ may fluoresce a clear apple-green under the Woods lamp in a darkened room.

17. Exposure to antibiotics provides _____ pressure, which makes the surviving bacteria more likely to be _____.

18. Bacteria that produce _____ are resistant to β-lactam antibiotics.

19. The _____ is the lowest concentration of the specific antimicrobial that can inhibit the growth of a given bacteria.

20. _____ refers to the dilution of the antimicrobial where a specific bacterium begins to show resistance.

EXERCISE 7.3: CROSSWORD PUZZLE: MICROBIOLOGY

Across
2 Unicellular fungi that reproduce by budding
3 A fungus that causes infections of the skin, hair, and nails
6 A disease that may be transmitted between animals and humans

Down
1 Describes microorganisms with complex nutritional requirements
4 An organism that can live and grow in the presence of oxygen
5 The lowest concentration of an antimicrobial agent that will inhibit the visible growth of a microorganism

EXERCISE 7.4: LABORATORY EXERCISE: QUADRANT STREAK METHOD FOR ISOLATING BACTERIA

Procedure:

1. Use a sterile bacteriologic loop to remove a small amount of the bacterial colony from the culture plate or a loopful from a broth culture.

2. *Optional:* Divide a plate into four quadrants by marking the bottom of the Petri dish with a black marker.

3. Hold the loop horizontally against the surface of the agar to avoid digging into the agar when streaking the inoculum.

4. Lightly streak the inoculating loop over one quarter (quadrant A) of the plate by using a back-and-forth motion; keep each streak separate.

5. Pass the loop through a flame, and allow it to cool.

6. Place the inoculating loop on the edge of quadrant A, and extend the streaks into quadrant B by using a back-and-forth motion.

7. Pass the loop through a flame, and allow it to cool.

8. Place the inoculating loop on the edge of quadrant B, and extend the streaks into quadrant C by using a back-and-forth motion.

9. Pass the loop through a flame, and allow it to cool.

10. Place the inoculating loop on the edge of quadrant C, and extend the streaks into quadrant D by using a back-and-forth motion.

EXERCISE 7.5: LABORATORY EXERCISE: INOCULATING AGAR SLANT AND BUTT

Procedure:

1. Use a sterile bacteriologic needle to remove a small amount of the bacterial colony from the culture plate or a loopful from a broth culture.

2. Stab the needle directly into the center of the agar, pushing the needle all the way down to the bottom of the tube.

3. Withdraw the inoculating needle through the same path in the agar.

4. Streak the slant by using a back-and-forth motion starting at the bottom of the slant.

EXERCISE 7.6: LABORATORY EXERCISE: GRAM STAIN PROCEDURE

Procedure:

1. Draw a circle with a wax pencil in the center of a clean glass slide.

2. Place a drop of saline in the circle on the slide, and transfer a small amount of the specimen, as appropriate (e.g., inoculating loop, swab, wire).

3. Allow the slide to air dry.

4. Heat fix the slide by passing it through a flame two or three times, specimen side up.

5. Place the slide over a staining rack.

6. Pour crystal violet over the sample area, and allow to sit for 30 seconds.

7. Rinse the slide with water.

8. Pour the iodine solution onto the area, and allow to sit for 30 seconds.

9. Rinse the slide with water.

10. Flood the slide with decolorizer until no more purple color washes off (generally about 10 seconds).

11. Rinse the slide with water.

12. Add the basic fuchsin (or safranin) to the sample area, and allow to sit for 30 seconds.

13. Rinse the slide with water.

14. Air dry the slide, or blot dry between sheets of paper towels.

15. Record the Gram stain results below.

GRAM STAIN RESULTS

Date collected _____ Patient ID _____ Species _____

Sample source _____ Gram stain reaction _____

Date collected _____ Patient ID _____ Species _____

Sample source _____ Gram stain reaction _____

Date collected _____ Patient ID _____ Species _____

Sample source _____ Gram stain reaction _____

EXERCISE 7.7: LABORATORY EXERCISE: POTASSIUM HYDROXIDE TEST

Procedure:

1. Place a loopful (or two, if necessary) of 3% potassium hydroxide (KOH) solution on a slide.

2. Transfer a generous quantity of surface growth from the culture to the drop of KOH.

3. Stir the specimen into the KOH drop with a loop; the loop is then lifted slowly and gently.

   a. After a maximum of 2 minutes of stirring (usually 30 seconds), gram-negative organisms develop a mucoid appearance and produce a sticky strand when the drop is lifted with the loop.

   b. If the organisms are gram positive, the mixture stays homogeneous and does not form a strand on lifting.

4. The reaction is recorded as gram negative (sticky strand and mucoid mass formed) or gram positive (no sticky strand or mucoid mass formed).

109

Procedure:

1. For direct sensitivity testing:

   a. Insert a sterile swab into a fresh urine sample collected by cystocentesis or catheterization.

2. For indirect sensitivity testing:

   a. Select four or five well-isolated colonies of the same morphologic type from an agar plate.

   b. Touch the top of each colony with a wire loop, and transfer the growth to a tube containing 0.5 to 1 mL of saline or broth.

      i. The turbidity of the bacterial suspensions should be equivalent to a MacFarland #5 standard.

   c. Within 15 minutes after preparing the suspension, dip a sterile cotton swab into the suspension, and rotate the swab several times, with pressure on the inside wall of the tube to remove excess inoculum from the swab.

3. Inoculate the Mueller-Hinton medium by streaking the swab horizontally across the entire surface of the medium; then rotate the plate 60 degrees, and inoculate again. Repeat, as needed, to ensure that the plate is evenly covered.

4. Use an antimicrobial disk dispenser or sterile forceps to place the antimicrobial disks on the inoculated agar surface.

   a. The disks should be no closer than 10 to 15 mm to the edge of the plate and sufficiently separated from each other by about 24 mm to avoid overlapping of the zones of inhibition.

5. Unless the disks were placed with a self-tamping dispenser, use a second sterile swab to gently press the antibiotic disks into the agar.

6. Incubate the plate aerobically at 37° C.

   a. Plates should be placed in the incubator within 15 minutes after placing the disks on the inoculated agar.

   b. Inoculated plates should be inverted before placing them in the incubator to keep condensation from forming on the surface of the agar.

7. After 18 to 24 hours of incubation, perform physical measurement of the inhibitory zones.

   a. Measure the diameter of each inhibition zone to the nearest millimeter (including the diameter of the disk) from the underside of the plate using calipers, a transparent ruler, or a template.

   b. If Mueller-Hinton agar with blood has been used, the zone size must be read from the top surface, with the lid of the plate removed.

8. Compare the measurement to a chart of inhibitory zones to determine the relative resistance of the bacterium to the antibiotics being tested.

9. Record results as resistant, intermediate, or susceptible for each antimicrobial tested.

Chart of Inhibitory Zones to Determine the Relative Resistance of the Bacterium to the Antibiotics Being Tested				
Antimicrobial Agent	Disk Content	Susceptible	Intermediate	Resistant
Amikacin	30 mg	≥17	15-16	≤14
Amoxicillin/clavulanic acid (staphylococci)	20/10 mg	≥20		≤19
Amoxicillin/clavulanic acid (other organisms)	20/10 mg	≥18	14-17	≤13 .
Ampicillin* (gram-negative enteric organisms)	10 mg	≥17	14-16	≤13
Ampicillin* (staphylococci)	10 mg	≥29		≤28
Ampicillin* (enterococci)	10 mg	≥17		≤16
Ampicillin* (streptococci)	10 mg	≥26	19-25	≤18
Cefazolin	30 mg	≥18	15-17	≤14
Ceftiofur (respiratory pathogens only)	30 mg	≥21	18-20	≤17
Cephalothin†	30 mg	≥18	15-17	≤14
Chloramphenicol	30 mg	≥18	13-17	≤12
Clindamycin‡	2 mg	≥21	15-20	≤14
Enrofloxacin	5 mg	≥23	17-22	≤13
Erythromycin	15 mg	≥23	14-22	≤13
Florfenicol	30 mg	≥19	15-18	≤14
Gentamicin	10 mg	≥15	13-14	≤12
Kanamycin	30 mg	≥18	14-17	≤13
Oxacillin§ (staphylococci)	1 mg	≥13	11-12	≤10
Penicillin G (staphylococci)	10 U	≥29		≤28
Penicillin G (enterococci)	10 U	≥15		≤14
Penicillin G (streptococci)	10 U	≥28	20-27	≤19
Penicillin/novobiocini	10 U/30 mg	≥18	15-17	≤14 .
Pirlimycin‖	2 mg	≥13		≤12
Rifampin	5 mg	≥20	17-19	≤16
Sulfonamides	250 or 300 mg	≥17	13-16	≤12
Tetracycline¶	30 mg	≥19	15-18	≤14
Ticarcillin (*Pseudomonas aeruginosa*)	75 mg	≥15		≤14
Ticarcillin (gram-negative enteric organisms)	75 mg	≥20	15-19	≤14
Tilmicosin	15 mg	≥14	11-13	≤10
Trimethoprim/sulfamethoxazole**	1.25/23.75 mg	≥16	11-15	≤10

*Ampicillin is used to test for susceptibility to amoxicillin and hetacillin.

†Cephalothin is used to test all first-generation cephalosporins, such as cephapirin and cefadroxil. Cefazolin should be tested separately with the gram-negative enteric organisms.

‡Clindamycin is used to test for susceptibility to clindamycin and lincomycin.

§Oxacillin is used to test for susceptibility to methicillin, nafcillin, and cloxacillin.

‖Available as an infusion product for treatment of bovine mastitis during lactation.

¶Tetracycline is used to test for susceptibility to chlortetracycline, oxytetracycline, minocycline, and doxycycline.

**Trimethoprim/sulfamethoxazole is used to test for susceptibility to trimethoprim/sulfadiazine and ormetoprim/ sulfadimethoxine.

EXERCISE 7.9: LABORATORY EXERCISE: CATALASE TEST

Procedure:

1. Place a small amount of material from an isolated colony on a blood agar plate on a microscope slide.

    a. Ensure that no agar is transferred with the colony.

2. Add 1 drop of catalase reagent (3% hydrogen peroxide).

3. Record as positive if gas bubbles are produced within 10 seconds.

4. Record as negative if no bubbles are produced within 10 seconds.

Date collected _____ Patient ID _____ Species _____

Sample source _____ Catalase reaction _____

Date collected _____ Patient ID _____ Species _____

Sample source _____ Catalase reaction _____

Date collected _____ Patient ID _____ Species _____

Sample source _____ Catalase reaction _____

EXERCISE 7.10: LABORATORY EXERCISE: DERMATOPHYTE TEST

Procedure:

1. Gently clean the skin lesion to remove some of the surface contamination.

2. Collect specimens from the lesion periphery.

    a. Pluck broken hair shafts and dry scale because these are most likely to contain viable organisms.

3. Push the specimens into and partially below the surface of the media.

4. Incubate the culture at room temperature with the cap or plate cover loosened; observe daily for growth.

5. At the first sign of color change, perform a wet prep and lactophenol cotton blue stain to confirm the presence of pathogenic forms.

Instructions: Find the words that are defined by the clues given below. The words may be located horizontally, vertically, or diagonally and may be reversed.

```
I  C  L  C  C  R  L  O  L  E  R  S  B  C  O
R  R  C  U  L  T  U  R  E  T  T  E  A  R  P
C  I  L  I  H  P  O  R  E  A  O  R  C  I  M
F  A  N  L  T  I  O  N  M  L  N  O  I  N  E
I  L  P  C  L  E  T  S  E  L  P  P  L  G  H
E  W  A  N  U  L  M  R  S  O  N  S  L  W  R
S  U  I  G  O  B  O  D  O  C  D  O  I  O  O
A  A  I  G  E  P  A  A  P  Y  T  C  L  R  T
D  A  B  L  S  L  H  T  H  L  D  S  S  M  T
I  A  I  O  E  A  L  I  I  G  R  A  C  P  I
X  O  D  Y  U  C  M  A  L  O  C  C  S  A  I
O  N  S  B  I  R  O  N  E  I  N  S  X  E  A
E  S  A  L  A  T  A  C  L  H  C  C  A  O  O
S  H  O  O  T  E  T  U  C  T  U  P  I  L  S
O  N  A  P  G  E  L  L  D  I  O  Z  I  H  R
```

ASCOSPORES	COCCI	INCUBATION	RHIZOID
BACILLI	CULTURETTE	MESOPHILE	RINGWORM
CAPNOPHILIC	ENDOSPORE	MICROAEROPHILIC	SABOURAUD
CATALASE	FLAGELLA	OXIDASE	THIOGLYCOLLATE

DTM Test Report

Date collected _____ Patient ID _____ Species _____

Observation Day	Date	Color Change Y/N?	Growth Y/N?	Microscopic Examination Results
1				
2				
3				
4				
5				
6				
7				
8				
9				
10				
11				
12				
13				
14				

DTM Test Report

Date collected _____ Patient ID _____ Species _____

Observation Day	Date	Color Change Y/N?	Growth Y/N?	Microscopic Examination Results
1				
2				
3				
4				
5				
6				
7				
8				
9				
10				
11				
12				
13				
14				

Microbiology Report

Date collected _____ Patient ID _____ Species _____

Sample type _____ Collection method _____

Culture media used _____

Bacteria morphology _____ Initial Gram reaction: _____

Results

Colony Characteristics

Size	
Pigment	
Density	
Elevation	
Form	
Texture	
Odor	
Hemolysis	

Additional Testing:	Result
Acid-fast stain	
Endosphore stain	
Catalase test	
Coagulase test	
Oxidase test	
C&S	

Presumptive identification: _____

Microbiology Report

Date collected _____ Patient ID _____ Species _____

Sample type _____ Collection method _____

Culture media used _____

Bacteria morphology _____ Initial Gram reaction: _____

Results

Colony Characteristics

Size	
Pigment	
Density	
Elevation	
Form	
Texture	
Odor	
Hemolysis	

Additional Testing:	Result
Acid-fast stain	
Endosphore stain	
Catalase test	
Coagulase test	
Oxidase test	
C&S	

Presumptive identification: _____

8 Parasitology

When you have completed this unit, you should be able to:

1. State the generalized life cycle of nematodes and trematodes.

2. List the common species of roundworms, hookworms, lungworms, and whipworms that affect domestic animals.

3. Discuss the life cycle of the canine heartworm.

4. Identify ova of common parasites of domestic animals.

5. Describe the life cycle of common cestodes.

6. Describe the life cycles of ticks.

7. Describe the general characteristics of organisms in the phylum Arthropoda.

8. List the commonly encountered species of fleas, ticks, mites, and lice that parasitize veterinary species.

9. Perform fecal analysis on samples from small and large animal patients.

EXERCISE 8.1: FILL-IN-THE-BLANK: PARASITOLOGY REVIEW

Instructions: Fill in each of the spaces provided with the missing word or words that complete the sentence.

1. Organisms in the phylum Nematoda are commonly called _____.

2. The developmental stages in the life cycle of a nematode are _____, _____, and _____.

3. A life cycle is considered _____ if no intermediate host is necessary for development to the infective stage.

4. The primary ascarids that infect puppies and kittens are _____, _____, and _____.

5. Adult *Dirofilaria immitis* are found within the _____, _____, and _____.

6. The prepatent period of *D. immitis* in dogs is approximately _____.

7. The _____ is the intermediate host for *D. immitis*.

8. The microfilariae of _____ nonpathogenic nematodes must be differentiated from those of *D. immitis*.

9. Tapeworms are dorsoventrally flattened and contain segments known as _____.

10. A dog or cat becomes infected with the tapeworm _____ by ingesting the flea intermediate host.

11. The intermediate hosts for *Taenia pisiformis* are _____ and _____.

12. The tapeworm _____ is the hydatid cyst tapeworm of dogs.

13. *Nanophyetus salmincola* is commonly referred to as the _____ of dogs.

14. The three primary phyla of parasitic protozoa are _____.

15. The term _____ refers to the motile, feeding stage of a protozoal parasite.

16. _____ is a protozoal parasite described as pear shaped and dorsoventrally flattened with four pairs of flagella.

17. Infection with _____ manifests as infertility, spontaneous abortion, and pyometra.

18. Cats infected with _____ generally only shed oocysts for less than 2 weeks for their entire life.

19. _____ are basophilic, pear-shaped trophozoites found in the red blood cells (RBCs) on stained blood smears.

20. The _____ are a group of obligate intracellular gram-negative bacteria and transmitted by arthropod or helminth vectors.

21. _____ can act as intermediate hosts for the common tapeworm, *Dipylidium caninum*.

22. The biting and chewing lice are in the order _____, and the sucking lice are in the order _____.

23. Infestation by larval dipterans is referred to as _____.

24. Immunodeficiency of the host is necessary for infestation with _____ mites to be clinically apparent.

25. _____ is a species of mite that lives in the external ear canal of dogs and cats.

EXERCISE 8.2: DEFINING KEY TERMS

Instructions: Define each term in your own words.

1. Definitive host

   _____

   _____

2. Prepatent period

   _____

   _____

3. Paratenic host

   _____

   _____

4. Pediculosis

   _____

   _____

5. Acariasis

   _____

   _____

6. Describe the method used to recover the ova of *Oxyuris*.

_____

_____

7. List the larval stages of trematodes.

_____

_____

8. List conditions under which a protozoal parasite might develop into a cyst.

_____

_____

_____

_____

EXERCISE 8.3: FILL-IN-THE-BLANK: COMMON PARASITES

Instructions: Complete the following chart.

Scientific Name	Common Name
Dogs	
Acanthocheilonema reconditum	
Ancylostoma caninum	
Pearsonema plica	
Dioctophyma renale	
Dirofilaria immitis	
Spirocerca lupi	
Thelazia californiensis	
Toxocara canis	
Trichuris vulpis	
Uncinaria stenocephala	
Diphyllobothrium species	
Cats	
Aelurostrongylus abstrusus	
Ancylostoma braziliense	
Ancylostoma tubaeforme	
Physaloptera species	
Spirocerca lupi	
Thelazia californiensis	
Toxascaris leonina	
Toxocara cati	
Trichuris serrata	
Echinococcus multilocularis	

Scientific Name	Common Name
Ruminants	
Bunostomum species	
Cooperia species	
Dictyocaulus filaria	
Dictyocaulus viviparus	
Gongylonema pulchrum	
Haemonchus species	
Marshallagia species	
Muellerius capillaris	
Nematodirus species	
Protostrongylus species	
Setaria cervi	
Strongyloides papillosus	
Thelazia gulosa	
Thelazia rhodesii	
Trichuris ovis	
Taenia saginata	
Horses	
Dictyocaulus arnfieldi	
Onchocerca cervicalis	
Oxyuris equi	
Parascaris equorum	
Setaria equina	
Strongyloides westeri	
Thelazia lacrymalis	
Pigs	
Ascaris suum	
Ascarops strongylina	
Hyostrongylus rubidus	
Metastrongylus elongatus	
Oesophagostomum dentatum	
Pigs	
Physocephalus sexalatus	
Stephanurus dentatus	
Trichinella spiralis	
Trichuris suis	

EXERCISE 8.4: WORD SEARCH: PARASITOLOGY

Instructions: Find the words that are defined by the clues given below. The words may be located horizontally, vertically, or diagonally and may be reversed.

```
T   O   K   C   A   A   H   A   C   I   X   O   A   T   E   S

A   O   O   S   E   T   I   O   Z   Y   H   C   A   T   C   M

E   A   A   O   N   C   O   S   T   C   Z   C   M   E   L   A

D   S   D   A   D   T   U   O   E   T   E   T   A   T   A   A

O   A   T   A   O   E   E   T   M   G   C   S   S   R   E   K

T   A   M   O   P   Z   D   L   I   Z   A   Y   T   I   T   T

A   I   I   I   A   P   O   O   C   C   O   I   O   L   O

M   S   C   Y   R   O   T   T   R   O   L   T   G   O   D   A

E   T   I   S   A   R   A   P   O   T   C   E   O   L   H   E

R   T   M   E   S   O   M   L   F   R   X   O   T   I   X   E

T   E   C   X   I   O   E   O   I   A   P   E   E   T   A   L

O   K   T   Z   T   I   N   O   L   O   S   O   L   D   S   I

A   C   T   H   E   X   A   C   A   N   T   H   M   O   G   H

D   I   T   T   O   L   G   O   R   P   P   A   I   E   C   H

O   R   C   A   S   C   A   R   I   D   S   S   G   S   H   S

N   A   T   O   O   Z   E   W   A   R   B   L   E   S   E   I
```

AMASTIGOTE	HEMOPROTOZOA	RICKETTSIA
ASCARID	HEXACANTH	SCOLEX
CESTODE	MICROFILARIA	TACHYZOITES
CUTICLE	NEMATODE	TREMATODE
ECTOPARASITE	OOCYST	WARBLES
ENDOPARASITE	PROGLOTTID	

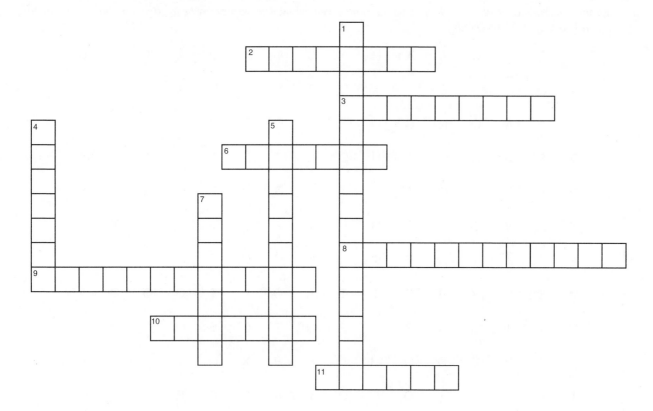

Across

2 Life cycle stage of trematodes that develops in the intermediate host
3 Organism commonly referred to as a fluke
6 Common name for the larva of some species of flies; often in fistulated subcutaneous sites
8 A parasite that resides within a host's tissues
9 A parasite that resides on the surface of its host
10 Infestation with larvae (maggots) of dipterans
11 The "head" of a cestode by which it attaches to its host

Down

1 Condition in which female organisms produce eggs that develop without fertilization
4 Outer layer or covering of epithelium
5 Segments that comprise the body of a cestode
7 Any of the nematodes of the Ascaridoidea family

Match the image on the left with the description on the right

1.
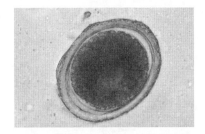

a. *Otodectes cyanotis*

2.
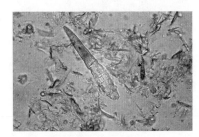

b. *Pearsonema plica*

3.
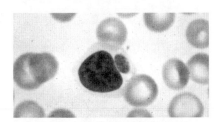

c. *Ancylostoma caninum*

4.
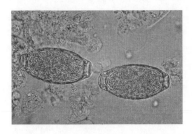

d. *Oxyuris equi*

5.
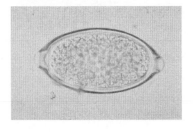

e. *Dioctophyma renale*

6.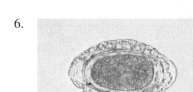

f. Taeniid ova

7.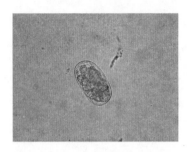

g. *Toxocara* species

8.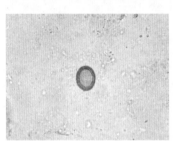

h. *Ehrlichia canis*

9.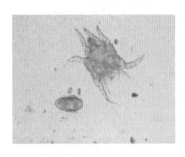

i. *Giardia*

10.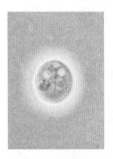

j. *Trichuris vulpis*

11.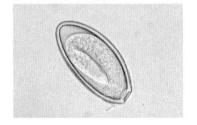

k. Adult *Demodex canis*

EXERCISE 8.7: LABORATORY EXERCISE: DIRECT SMEAR OF FECES

Procedure:

1. Dip the applicator stick into the feces specimen. (Only a small amount should adhere to the stick.)

2. Place 1 drop of saline on a slide.

3. Mix the feces specimen with saline to produce a homogeneous emulsion that is clear enough to read newsprint through it. (A common mistake is to make the smear too thick.)

4. Place the coverslip over the emulsion.

5. Examine the slide at $100\times$ and $400\times$ magnification for eggs, cysts, trophozoites, and larvae.

Optional: To demonstrate diagnostic features of protozoa, add 1 drop of Lugol iodine:

1. To make a 5% Lugol stock solution, add 5 g of iodine crystals to 10 g of potassium iodide/100 mL distilled water.

2. Store solution in an amber bottle away from light.

3. Dilute one part 5% Lugol stock solution to five parts distilled water to make a staining solution.

EXERCISE 8.8: LABORATORY EXERCISE: SIMPLE FECAL FLOTATION

Procedure:

1. Place approximately 2 to 5 g of the feces specimen in the paper cup.

2. Add 30 mL of flotation solution.

3. Using a tongue depressor, mix the feces specimen to produce an evenly suspended emulsion.

4. If using cheesecloth, bend the sides of the cup to form a spout, and cover the top with cheesecloth squares while pouring the suspension into the shell vial. If using a metal strainer, pour the suspension through the metal strainer into another cup, and fill the shell vial with the filtered solution.

5. Fill the shell vial to form a convex dome (meniscus) at the rim. Do not overfill the vial. Fresh solution can be used to form this dome.

6. Place a coverslip on top of the filled shell vial.

7. Allow the coverslip to remain undisturbed for 10 to 20 minutes.

8. Pick the coverslip straight up, and place it on a glass slide, fluid side down.

9. Systematically examine the surface under the coverslip at $100\times$ magnification.

EXERCISE 8.9: LABORATORY EXERCISE: CENTRIFUGAL FLOTATION

Procedure:

1. Prepare a fecal emulsion using 2 to 5 g of feces and 30 mL of flotation solution.

2. Strain the emulsion through cheesecloth or a tea strainer into the centrifuge tube. (Suspending a funnel over the tube facilitates filling the tube.)

3. Fill the tube to create a positive meniscus with flotation solution.

4. Place a coverslip on top of the tube.

5. Create a balance tube of equal weight, containing another sample or water.

6. Place the tubes in the centrifuge buckets, and weigh them on a balance. You may add water to the buckets to make them have equal weight.

7. Centrifuge the tubes for 5 minutes at 400 to 650 g (–1500 rpm).

8. Remove the coverslips from the tubes by lifting them straight up, and place them on a slide.

9. Systematically examine the slides at 100× magnification.

EXERCISE 8.10: LABORATORY EXERCISE: FECAL SEDIMENTATION

Procedure:

1. Mix 2 to 5 g of feces in a cup with 30 mL of water.

2. Strain the fecal suspension through cheesecloth or a tea strainer into a 50-mL conical centrifuge tube. (Suspending a funnel over the tube facilitates filling the tube.)

3. Wash the sample with water until the tube is filled.

4. Allow the tube to sit undisturbed for 15 to 30 minutes.

5. Decant the supernatant off, and resuspend the sediment in water.

6. Repeat steps 4 and 5 two more times.

7. Decant the supernatant without disturbing the sediment.

8. Using a pipette, mix the sediment, and transfer an aliquot to a slide.

9. Place a coverslip over the sediment, and systematically examine the slide with 100× magnification.

10. Repeat steps 8 and 9 until all sediment has been examined.

EXERCISE 8.11: LABORATORY EXERCISE: CELLOPHANE TAPE PREPARATION

Procedure:

1. Place adhesive tape in a loop around one end of the tongue depressor with the adhesive side facing out.

2. Press the tape firmly against the skin around the anus of the animal.

3. Place 1 drop of water on the slide. Undo the loop of tape, and stick the tape to the slide, allowing the water to spread out under the tape.

4. Examine the taped area of the slide microscopically for the presence of pinworm eggs.

EXERCISE 8.12: LABORATORY EXERCISE: BAERMANN TECHNIQUE

Procedure:

1. Construct a Baermann apparatus by fastening the ring to the ring stand. Attach 3 to 4 inches of rubber tubing to the narrow portion of the funnel. Ensure that there is a good seal (tubing can be glued on). Place the funnel in the ring. Place the wire screen in the top portion of the funnel to support the feces specimen. Put several layers of cheesecloth or KimWipes over the wire screen. Place the pinch clamps at the end of the rubber tubing, and check, using water, to ensure a tight seal. Put 30 to 50 g of feces on top of the KimWipes, and fill the funnel with warm water (not hot) to a level above the fecal sample.

2. An alternative method, which is more practical in the clinical practice setting, is to use long-stem, plastic champagne glasses with hollow stems. The fecal samples are wrapped in several layers of KimWipes to simulate a tea bag. The fecal pouch is then set in the glass. Fill the glass with warm water to a level above the fecal sample.

3. Allow the apparatus to remain undisturbed for a minimum of 1 hour and up to 24 hours.

4. Collect the fluid in the rubber tubing (stem of the glass) and transfer to a Petri dish or centrifuge tube.

5. Examine the Petri dish for larvae by using a stereo-microscope, or centrifuge the solution to pellet the larvae. Remove the supernatant from the centrifuge tube, and place the pellet on a microscope slide.

6. Examine the slide for larvae, and identify them. The slide can be passed over the flame of a Bunsen burner several times to kill the larvae in an extended position before identification.

EXERCISE 8.13: LABORATORY EXERCISE: BUFFY COAT SMEAR

Procedure:

1. Fill the hematocrit tube with the blood sample, and plug one end with sealant.

2. Centrifuge for 5 minutes. Use the file to etch the glass below the buffy coat. (The buffy coat is located in the middle of the centrifuged sample between RBCs and plasma.)

3. Snap the tube by applying pressure opposite the etched spot.

4. Take the end of the tube containing the buffy coat and plasma and tap the buffy coat onto a glass slide with a small amount of plasma. If too much plasma is released, use a clean KimWipe to wipe away the excess.

5. Apply a clean slide over the buffy coat, and rapidly pull the two slides across each other in opposite directions.

6. Allow the slides to air dry, and stain with Romanowsky stain.

7. After staining, apply the mounting medium and a coverslip.

8. Examine the slides microscopically at 400× and 1000× magnification.

EXERCISE 8.14: LABORATORY EXERCISE: MODIFIED KNOTT'S TECHNIQUE

Procedure:

1. Mix 1 mL of blood with 9 mL of 2% formalin in a centrifuge tube. Agitate the tube, and mix well.

2. Centrifuge the tube at 1500 rpm for 5 minutes.

3. Pour off the supernatant, and add 1 to 2 drops of methylene blue stain to the pellet at the bottom of the tube.

4. Using a pipette, mix the stain and sediment, and transfer the mixture to a glass slide.

5. Apply a coverslip and examine the sediment microscopically for microfilariae at 100× and 400× magnification.

127

Parasitology Report Form

Patient name: _____ Date: _____

Species: _____ Breed: _____ Age: _____ Gender: _____

Collection date/time: _____ Collection method: _____

Test(s) Performed	Result

Parasitology Report Form

Patient name: _____ Date: _____

Species: _____ Breed: _____ Age: _____ Gender: _____

Collection date/time: _____ Collection method: _____

Test(s) Performed	Result

9 Cytology

LEARNING OBJECTIVES

When you have completed this unit, you should be able to:

1. Describe sample collection techniques and collect cytology samples.

2. List and describe the methods that can be used to prepare cytology samples for evaluation.

3. Prepare cytology samples for microscopic examination.

4. Identify normal and common abnormal cells in cytology preparations.

EXERCISE 9.1: DEFINING KEY TERMS

Instructions: Define each term in your own words.

1. Centesis

   _____

2. Pleomorphism

   _____

3. Exudate

   _____

4. Anisokaryosis

   _____

5. Wave motion

   _____

EXERCISE 9.2: FILL-IN-THE-BLANK AND SHORT ANSWER: CYTOLOGY REVIEW

Instructions: Answer the following questions and fill in each of the spaces provided with the missing word or words that complete the sentence.

1. Unless the samples are from a moist lesion, swabs must be moistened with _____ before samples are collected.

2. Making multiple imprints from different layers of an external lesion is referred to as _____ preparation.

3. To ensure adequate fixation of histology samples, slabs of tissue no more than _____ wide should be placed in fluid-tight jars containing formalin at approximately _____ times the specimen's volume.

4. The _____, also called the needle spread technique, is ideal for the preparation of viscous samples.

5. Samples with low cellularity and small volume should be prepared with the _____ technique.

6. Prepared cytology slides should remain in fixative for _____ minutes before staining.

7. In fluid samples, total nucleated cell counts (TNCCs) of greater than _____ is a common finding with inflammation.

8. Suppurative inflammation is characterized by the presence of greater than _____ % of the TNCC.

9. _____ appears as a nucleus that appears swollen and ragged without an intact nuclear membrane and with reduced staining intensity.

10. _____ represents slow cell death (aging) and refers to a small, condensed, dark nucleus.

11. Hyperplasia with no criteria of malignancy present in the nucleus of the cells is described as _____.

12. Cells that display at least three abnormal nuclear configurations are identified as _____.

13. Epithelial cell tumors are also referred to as _____ or _____.

14. Mesenchymal cell tumors are also referred to as _____.

15. When greater than 15% of a cytology sample is composed of macrophages, the sample is classified as _____ or _____.

16. A sample characterized by the presence of large numbers of cells with an eccentrically located nucleus and prominent perinuclear clear zone most likely indicates a _____.

17. Yeasts, squamous epithelial cells, and _____ organisms are commonly isolated from ear swabs and may not indicate pathology.

18. In a normal lymph node, the predominant cell type is the _____.

19. Epithelial cells that are angular in appearance and have no nuclei or that contain pyknotic nuclei are described as _____.

20. Reactive lymph nodes contain predominantly small, mature lymphocytes as well as _____, lymphoblasts, and intermediate lymphocytes.

21. Plasma cells containing secretory vesicles of immunoglobulin are described as _____.

22. _____ cells line the body cavities.

23. A fluid sample with a high fat content and large number of mature lymphocytes is described as _____.

24. Normal peritoneal and pleural fluids have less than _____ nucleated cells/μL.

25. List the nuclear criteria of malignancy.

_____

_____

_____

_____

_____

26. Differentiate among samples from epithelial cell tumors, mesenchymal tumors, and discrete round cell tumors on the basis of their overall cellularity and exfoliative characteristics.

_____

_____

_____

_____

_____

_____

_____

_____

27. List the cell types that may be present in vaginal cytology samples.

_____

_____

_____

_____

_____

_____

28. List evaluations that may be performed on semen samples.

_____

_____

_____

_____

EXERCISE 9.3: WORD SEARCH: CYTOLOGY

Instructions: Find the words that are defined by the clues given below. The words may be located horizontally, vertically, or diagonally and may be reversed.

```
I   M   K   E   P   L   C   M   I   T   M   N   T   D   E   S   O
I   N   S   V   P   A   E   Y   I   I   D   R   L   A   U   K   R
A   E   A   M   A   M   T   T   R   A   N   S   U   D   A   T   E
P   B   R   Y   R   O   S   U   I   N   T   U   Y   R   A   S   N
P   D   C   S   A   T   S   I   S   O   N   K   Y   P   O   N   T
A   O   O   S   C   Y   A   C   H   O   C   O   O   C   H   G   E
E   O   M   E   E   C   K   I   O   P   R   R   A   A   D   I   V
O   S   A   I   N   O   A   E   E   R   R   I   M   A   E   N   I
E   T   L   V   T   I   E   X   H   T   N   O   A   G   A   E   T
C   S   I   S   E   T   N   E   C   O   N   I   M   O   D   B   A
R   U   G   I   S   S   X   I   T   I   S   E   F   O   O   H   R
O   N   N   L   I   I   R   S   C   A   S   E   H   I   E   O   U
E   I   A   E   S   H   S   R   L   T   D   G   R   R   E   L   P
R   N   N   T   E   M   A   P   U   E   A   U   C   R   A   D   P
P   Y   T   O   I   C   O   X   U   P   S   E   X   N   M   M   U
M   C   E   E   T   E   V   I   T   A   X   I   F   E   M   L   S
T   M   R   X   M   E   U   R   S   R   P   A   N   Y   S   A   P
```

ABDOMINOCENTESIS   HISTIOCYTOMA   PLEOMORPHISM
BENIGN   KARYORRHEXIS   PYKNOSIS
CARCINOMA   MALIGNANT   SARCOMA
CORNIFIED   NEOPLASIA   SUPPURATIVE
EXUDATE   PARACENTESIS   TRANSUDATE
FIXATIVE

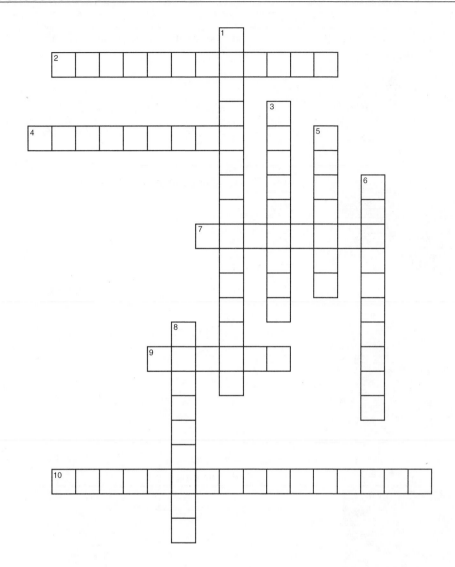

Across

2 Fragmentation of a cell nucleus
4 Describes tumors of epithelial cell origin
7 A tumor arising from melanocytes of the skin or other organs
9 Used to describe a tumor or growth that is not malignant
10 Paracentesis of the abdomen

Down

1 Removal of fluid from the thoracic cavity
3 Generic term to describe any growth; often used to describe a tumor, which may be malignant or benign
5 Any cancer arising from cells of the connective tissues
6 An effusion characterized by low protein concentration and low total nucleated cell counts
8 Act of puncturing a body cavity or organ with a hollow needle to draw out fluid

1.

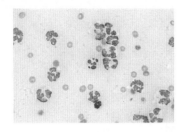

  a. Pyogranulomatous inflammation

2.

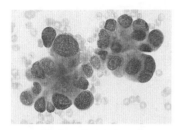

  b. Septic inflammation

3.

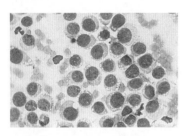

  c. *Malassezia* species

4.

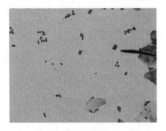

  d. Sarcoma

5.

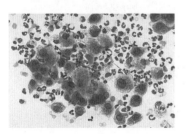

  e. Transmissible venereal tumor

6.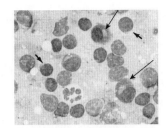

f. Suppurative inflammation

7.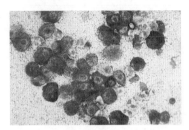

g. Mast cell tumor

8.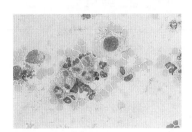

h. Plasma cells in a hyperplastic lymph node

9.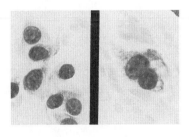

i. Eosinophilic inflammation

10.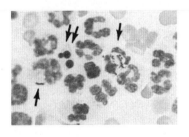

j. Lung carcinoma

EXERCISE 9.6: FILL-IN-THE-BLANK: EFFUSIONS

Instructions: Complete the following chart.

	1. _____	**Exudate**	**Modified Transudate**
Amount of fluid	Large	Variable	Variable
Color	Clear, colorless, or red tinged	2. _____	Variable; usually clear
Protein	<3.0 g/dL	3. _____	2.5-7.5 g/dL
TNCC	4. _____	>5000/μL	1000-7000/μL
Cell types	Mixture of monocytes, macrophages, lymphocytes, mesothelial cells	5. _____	6. _____

EXERCISE 9.7: LABORATORY EXERCISE: FINE-NEEDLE BIOPSY ASPIRATION PROCEDURE

Procedure:

1. Stabilize the mass.

2. Insert the needle into the mass.

3. Retract the syringe plunger to create negative pressure.

4. Redirect the needle several times.

   a. Do not exit the mass.

   b. Maintain negative pressure.

5. Remove the needle from the mass.

6. Remove the syringe from the needle.

7. Fill the syringe with air.

8. Reattach the needle.

9. Gently force the sample from the needle onto a clean slide.

10. Air dry, fix, and stain.

EXERCISE 9.8: LABORATORY EXERCISE: FINE-NEEDLE BIOPSY NONASPIRATION PROCEDURE

Procedure:

The procedure for this is the same as that for the aspiration procedure EXCEPT that just the needle or a needle or syringe with the syringe plunger removed is used.

1. Stabilize the mass.

2. Insert the needle into the mass.

3. Redirect the needle several times.

   a. Do not exit the mass.

   b. Maintain negative pressure.

4. Remove the needle from the mass.

   a. Remove the syringe from the needle.

5. Fill the syringe with air.

6. Reattach the needle.

7. Gently force the sample from the needle onto a clean slide.

8. Air dry, fix, and stain.

EXERCISE 9.9: LABORATORY EXERCISE: COMPRESSION SMEAR

Procedure:

Use a sample collected by fine-needle biopsy.

1. Transfer the sample to a clean slide near the frosted edge and toward the middle of the slide.

2. Add a second slide perpendicular to the first.

   a. Place the second slide on top of the drop of sample with the frosted edge facing down and close to the sample.

   b. Allow the sample to spread for a few seconds.

3. Using a smooth single motion, pull slide #2 (the top one) evenly across the bottom slide.

4. Air dry, fix, and stain slide #2.

EXERCISE 9.10: LABORATORY EXERCISE: MODIFIED COMPRESSION SMEAR

Procedure:

Use a sample collected by fine-needle biopsy.

1. Transfer the sample to a clean slide near the frosted edge and toward the middle of the slide.

2. Add a second slide perpendicular to the first.

   a. Place the second slide on top of the drop of sample with the frosted edge facing down and the sample near the middle of the slide.

   b. Allow the sample to spread for a few seconds.

3. Using a smooth single motion, twist the two slides in opposite directions.

4. Lift the top slide straight up.

5. Air dry, fix, and stain the top slide.

EXERCISE 9.11: LABORATORY EXERCISE: LINE SMEAR

Procedure:

Use a sample collected by fine-needle biopsy.

1. Transfer the sample to a clean slide near the frosted edge.

2. Use a second slide at an angle. Back the edge of the slide into the drop of sample.

3. Allow the sample to spread along the edge of the slide.

4. Use the second slide to push the sample across the slide.

5. STOP abruptly before the sample makes a feathered edge.

6. Pick the second slide straight up.

7. Air dry, fix, and stain slide #1.

EXERCISE 9.12: LABORATORY EXERCISE: WEDGE FILM

Procedure:

Use a sample collected by fine-needle biopsy.

1. Transfer the sample to a clean slide near the frosted edge.

2. Use a second slide at an angle. Back the edge of the slide into the drop of sample.

3. Allow the sample to spread along the edge of the slide.

4. Use the second slide to push the sample across the full length of the slide. The result is a feathered edge.

   a. To make the smear longer, lower the angle on the top slide.

   b. To make the smear shorter, increase the angle of the top slide.

5. Air dry, fix, and stain.

138

EXERCISE 9.13: LABORATORY EXERCISE: STARFISH SMEAR

Procedure:

Use a sample collected by fine-needle biopsy.

1. Transfer the sample to the center of a clean slide.

2. Use the tip of a needle to "drag" the sample outward from the center.

3. Vary the length and direction of each drag through the sample.

4. Air dry, fix, and stain.

EXERCISE 9.14: LABORATORY EXERCISE: SCRAPING

Procedure:

1. Use a scalpel blade to expose a fresh edge of the tissue.

2. Thoroughly blot the tissue.

3. Hold the blade at a 90-degree angle and scrape across the tissue.

4. Spread the sample onto a clean slide in a smooth motion.

    a. If the sample appears thick on the slide, make a compression smear from it.

5. Air dry, fix, and stain.

EXERCISE 9.15: LABORATORY EXERCISE: PUNCH BIOPSY

Procedure:

1. Gently rotate the biopsy punch in one direction until the punch blade has sectioned the tissue.

    a. Back-and-forth rotation increases the likelihood of specimen damage from shearing forces.

2. Grasp the margin of the tissue with a pair of fine forceps, or flush the tissue onto a small piece of wooden tongue depressor.

3. Allow the tissue to dry onto the tongue depressor.

4. Place the tissue with the attached tongue depressor "splint" into a formalin jar, specimen side down.

EXERCISE 9.16: LABORATORY EXERCISE: TOUCH IMPRINT

Procedure:

1. Expose a fresh edge on a small piece of tissue.

2. Thoroughly blot the tissue.

    a. Blot until the tissue is free of "juiciness."

3. Touch the tissue repeatedly in rows in single file or monolayers on a clean slide.

    a. Repeat the blotting, as needed.

4. Air dry, fix, and stain.

EXERCISE 9.17: LABORATORY EXERCISE: TZANCK PREP

Procedure:

1. Number four clean slides.

2. Touch the slide to the lesion on the patient as follows:

    a. Slide #1: Touch the slide to the unprepped lesion.

        i. You may first lightly wipe the lesion with saline.

    b. Slide #2: Prep, gently debride, and lightly clean the lesion, and touch the slide to the lesion.

    c. Slide #3: Fully debride the lesion, removing any scabs, and imprint the exposed area.

    d. Slide #4: Imprint the bottom of the scab.

3. Air dry, fix, and stain.

EXERCISE 9.18: LABORATORY EXERCISE: SWAB

Procedure:

1. Premoisten a swab with saline.

    a. A rayon swab, rather than a cotton swab, may be needed.

    b. A sterile swab may be needed.

2. Place the premoistened swab into the cavity.

3. Roll the swab in a single stroke in layers down the length of a clean slide.

4. Make two or three rows.

5. Air dry, fix, and stain.

Cytology Report

Patient name: _____ Date: _____

Species: _____ Breed: _____ Age: _____ Gender: _____

Sample type: _____ Collection method: _____

Preparation method: _____ Stain: _____

Results:

_____

_____

_____

_____

_____

_____

_____

For Fluid Samples:

Volume: _____

Color: _____

Protein: _____

TNCC: _____

Cytology Report

Patient name: _____ Date: _____

Species: _____ Breed: _____ Age: _____ Gender: _____

Sample type: _____ Collection method: _____

Preparation method: _____ Stain: _____

Results:

_____

_____

_____

_____

_____

_____

_____

_____

For Fluid Samples:

Volume: _____

Color: _____

Protein: _____

TNCC: _____

Cytology Report

Patient name: _____ Date: _____

Species: _____ Breed: _____ Age: _____ Gender: _____

Sample type: _____ Collection method: _____

Preparation method: _____ Stain: _____

Results:

_____

_____

_____

_____

_____

_____

_____

For Fluid Samples:

Volume: _____

Color: _____

Protein: _____

TNCC: _____

Cytology Report

Patient name: _____ Date: _____

Species: _____ Breed: _____ Age: _____ Gender: _____

Sample type: _____ Collection method: _____

Preparation method: _____ Stain: _____

Results:

_____

_____

_____

_____

_____

_____

_____

For Fluid Samples:

Volume: _____

Color: _____

Protein: _____

TNCC: _____